Liz Hodgkinson has been a newspaper and magazine journalist since 1967, specializing for the last few years in the health field. She has written many books including *Smile Therapy*, *Addictions*, *Sex Is Not Compulsory*, *Unholy Matrimony* and *The Alexander Technique*.

By the same author

LIZ HODGKINSON

HOW TO BANISH CELLULITE FOREVER

GRAFTON BOOKS

A Division of the Collins Publishing Group

LONDON GLASGOW
TORONTO SYDNEY AUCKLAND

Grafton Books
A Division of the Collins Publishing Group
8 Grafton Street, London W1X 3LA

A Grafton Paperback Original 1989
Copyright © Liz Hodgkinson 1989

ISBN 0-586-20601-9

Illustrations by Lorna Turpin
Printed and bound in Great Britain by
Collins, Glasgow

Set in Electra

ACKNOWLEDGEMENTS

I should particularly like to thank aromatherapists Patricia Davis and Frances Clifford for expert help in preparing this book. Thanks are also due to nutritionist Celia Wright, who first opened my eyes to the problem of cellulite, and to masseuse Clare Maxwell-Hudson, for valuable information on the many benefits of massage.

CONTENTS

PROLOGUE

Like many thousands of other women I have been plagued with ugly bumps and bulges on my thighs for most of my adult years.

It is not too much of an exaggeration to say that these nasty bulges have blighted my life. While they have never been life-threatening or a serious health risk, their all-too-obvious presence has meant that I've never really been able to wear tight jeans, shorts, short skirts, tracksuits or leggings. At least, I always felt I looked a complete fright in anything figure-hugging or leg-revealing. I've never felt comfortable in either bikinis or swimming costumes, and have not allowed anybody to take pictures of me on the beach. During the days of skintight, flared trousers, the ones supposedly in my size simply wouldn't accommodate my thighs. It may sound amusing now, but it was very upsetting at the time to a would-be slick chick.

The problem has been one that only I worried about or took seriously. Other people who knew about my hidden horrors just laughed, and could not understand my pre-occupation and worry about something so apparently trivial.

My close friends would go out of their way to assure me that I looked perfectly normal, very nice in fact.

But I was not reassured. The 'perfectly normal' appearance was only possible because I went to great lengths (literally) to hide the bumps and bulges. I always wore long skirts, baggy trousers and high-heeled shoes, and took a lot of care over hair and make-up so that attention would be diverted from the guilty secret – the overstuffed sausages I possessed instead of proper, long, slender thighs.

For a long time, I concluded that my horrible thighs must be just an unfortunate genetic inheritance I could do little about, such as a huge nose or receding chin might be. And yet I knew I hadn't always had such legs. Pictures of me as a child show me with perfectly slim, straight thighs. The acres of dimpled lard descended in late adolescence when I was about fifteen or sixteen and then simply stayed there, weighing me down and making me extremely self-conscious.

But at the back of my mind I never really accepted that nature had intended me to have these lumps and bulges. If so, then she was monstrously unfair, as I couldn't help noticing that not every young woman had them. Although the bulges and dimples were common enough, I could see for myself that they were not an inevitable accompaniment to womanhood. What's more, I wasn't generally fat or over-weight. My weight-for-height has always been exactly right according to the tables that are frequently published. All my adult life my thighs have looked as though they belonged to somebody else. I had to put up with fat thighs on an otherwise thin body.

But it wasn't really the girth of my thighs that upset me so much. If they had been merely fat, or well-built, I could have tolerated them more. It was the pockets of fat, the bulges, the jodhpurs, or 'love handles' as they are known in America, that I hated so much. The general appearance was as if somebody had forgotten to say when.

Over the years I tried everything I could to get rid of the bulges and regain the slim, shapely thighs of my pre-adolescence. In fact, most of us with this problem do 'try everything' to slim them down a bit and make them a little more presentable. I went on stringent diets. I did huge amounts of exercise. I went to health farms and submitted myself to saunas, starvation regimes, and endless pummell-ing and pounding. I went on marathon walks, gave up butter and dairy produce, became vegetarian. I stopped drinking and smoking. I took up yoga, and attempted to contort myself into unlikely positions. As I did so, I could feel the bulges stopping me from attaining the correct postures. It felt like having several bean bags in the way. The only problem was, the bean bags were inside my skin.

While all this effort ensured that I became extremely thin everywhere else, the thigh bulges stayed firmly in place, apparently unbudgeable. Of course, I was a sucker for every 'slim your thighs' book on the market. My friends, knowing about my – to them – needless sensitivity, would buy me thigh-reducing books for Christmas. I also tried the many patent creams which were advertised as having the ability to disperse fat from 'problem areas' such as hips and thighs. Thigh-reducing treatments are still a huge industry – along with all other slimming products.

Needless to say, these creams and lotions didn't even begin

to work. Nor did any of the special 'thigh-whittling' exercises which the books recommended. More than ever I became convinced that Mother Nature had doled out these hideous thighs to me as some obscure punishment, to remind me not to get too uppity. I couldn't think what I had done to deserve them, though. Finally, in desperation, I considered plastic surgery or liposuction, where excess fat is vacuumed out of thighs and buttocks.

One look at the before-and-after pictures, though, decided me against this operation. For while the patients had undoubtedly lost inches, *all their bulges and dimples were still there*. Even that drastic measure didn't result in straight, unbumpy thighs.

It was a great relief to me to learn that cosmetic surgery wouldn't solve my problem, because I am a terrible coward and cannot stand any kind of physical pain. Apart from that, these operations are always so very expensive, and can be dangerous.

Now though, all that agonizing, all that hatred directed against my unlovely thighs, is in the past. These days I do not have any lumps or bulges at all. My legs above the knee no longer have an overstuffed look but are the slim, straight limbs I have always coveted. Wonder of wonders, I can now wear tight jeans, tracksuits, bikinis and short skirts if I want to. I am no longer self-conscious about appearing on the beach. I have, at last, been able to accept my thighs as part of me rather than an alien graft, which was how I regarded them before.

When I survey my thighs nowadays I can hardly believe they are mine. In fact, it all seems so much like a dream come true that I often wonder if I will wake up one morning and find that the stuffed mattresses have come back. So far, I'm glad to say, they haven't.

I can't begin to estimate what a difference having thin thighs has made. My self-confidence and self-esteem have shot up and my former self-consciousness has disappeared. I'm quite happy now to wear a leotard or leggings, to reveal my thighs instead of wanting to cover them up and hide them. It's not nice to be desperately ashamed of a part of your body, and my relief at having really quite nice thighs, after two decades of misery over completely unaesthetic ones, is overwhelming.

So what have I done to achieve this miracle? It's quite simple. I came to learn that these bumps and bulges which had so clouded my adult years were not an inherited tendency, nor were they 'womanly curves'. And they were not, in the strict sense of the word, fat.

The dimpled bulges were, in fact, deposits of cellulite, toxic wastes which often accumulate in female fatty tissues and which the body is unable to expel by any usual means.

Yes, I can hear you laughing already. We all know that the term 'cellulite' has similar connotations to flying saucers, spoon bending and fairies at the bottom of the garden – one of the hardy annuals trotted out by newspapers and magazines when they can't think of anything else to write about. And those who consider themselves sophisticated tend to take the attitude that if you believe in cellulite you'll believe in anything.

Theories about cellulite have long been relegated to the cranky, bogus end of the health and beauty scene. The

British medical profession has, in recent years, done its best to discredit the notion that poisonous waste can somehow deposit itself on female thighs. And I must admit that when you first hear the idea it does sound pretty implausible. Because the thing is, men don't get cellulite – it's a female-only problem.

Most doctors maintain that there is no such thing as cellulite, no such thing as a special kind of fat which only women have. If some women do have these bulges on their thighs, well, they just have to learn to put up with them, that's all. Thigh bulges are just tough luck, and really nothing whatever to worry about. They're not an *illness*, for goodness' sake, most doctors will tell you.

The popular idea of cellulite is that it is a pure invention of cosmetic companies and slimming magazines who want to sell their products and periodicals, and which women are daft enough to believe. Why, even the word itself doesn't exist in the English language. It is a French import, rather like *ooh là là* or *zut alors* – and with about as much meaning for the medical profession. Because we in Britain and America largely don't accept the concept of cellulite we have no word for it. Officially, medically speaking, there's no such thing.

I used to think myself that the idea of cellulite was pure nonsense, something dreamed up by get-rich-quick merchants to play on women's deep-seated fears and insecurities. After all, I didn't want to be considered gullible and naïve. I regarded myself as a sophisticated and cynical journalist, not readily able to have the wool pulled over my eyes.

But when I heard about a treatment which was guaranteed

to get rid of cellulite, I decided to give it a try. The treatment consisted of a combination of a detoxifying diet, brushing yourself with a hard, scratchy brush made of Mexican cactus, and having aromatherapy oils massaged into the bulges. A few weeks of this regime, I was assured, would make all my cellulite deposits go.

I checked out that the treatments could do no harm, and also that the people offering them were genuine, rather than conwomen just after my money. When I was satisfied on both counts, I became my own guinea pig. I must say, though, that it was in a spirit of the profoundest scepticism that I made my first visit to a nearby aromatherapist. How, I wondered, could her treatments work when everything else, including the most austere of diets, had done nothing to shift the lumps and bumps? And how could she be so sure that cellulite existed, when all the doctors assured me time and again that it was a load of rubbish?

Well, all I can say is that the treatments did work – wonderfully. Nobody was more surprised than I when the lumps and bumps which had been there for two decades, seemingly unshiftable, finally began to soften and eventually disappear altogether. So I wasn't meant to have those bulges after all. Mother Nature hadn't played a cruel trick on me. The deposits were simply waste material that for a long time I hadn't been able to get rid of – and now I had succeeded. The tape measure and other people's comments proved beyond all possible doubt that the ghastly bulges had at long last vanished.

Now when I meet people in the street who haven't seen me for a long time they simply don't recognize me. When they realize who I am their first comment is always: 'Haven't you lost a lot of weight?'

Yet I haven't, really. I've only lost the bulges. The odd thing is that I look far thinner, even in long, bunchy skirts. Some people have told me I now walk differently, more like a fairy than an elephant, as previously. I look lighter, I'm told. And all because the thigh bulges have gone. Because they are not there any more I look like a different person altogether.

Once I embarked on the treatments I investigated the phenomenon of cellulite as thoroughly and scientifically as possible. It's not always easy, making a study of something you have been told categorically doesn't exist. But, I reasoned, that didn't stop Columbus, Galileo and all the other pioneers who have challenged the prevailing orthodoxy. You may say that discovering cellulite isn't as important as knowing whether the world is round, or whether the earth moves round the sun or vice versa. But to me it is. While I can be perfectly happy without any knowledge of geography or astronomy, it is difficult to be completely content with hideous thighs you have to view every single day of your life whether you like it or not.

Anyway, my researches have proved to me that, whatever the doctors say, there is such a thing as cellulite, that it is not the same as ordinary fat, and that there are treatments which will banish it for ever. Doctors don't know everything these days, any more than they ever did.

I believe now that cellulite is an indication of a chronic and possibly quite serious health problem. The deposits are no more supposed to be there than a wart, a verruca or an ingrowing toenail are supposed to be there. The presence of cellulite is an indication that not all is well inside your body.

When I made up my mind to try, finally, to get rid of my lumps and bumps, I enlisted the aid of a professional therapist. In my case this was necessary, as I was still extremely wary of accepting that cellulite existed, and I had to be persuaded by treatments that would work. Also, initially, I knew nothing about the subject, and had to gain information gradually. But it is perfectly possible to treat cellulite all by yourself once you understand what the problem is and why it affects only women.

There is no harm that can come to you from the treatments described in this book, and they have a huge advantage over 'miracle cures' in that they actually do work.

The anti-cellulite programme, in common with most worthwhile things in life, takes quite a bit of dedication and motivation. There's no pill you can swallow to make the cellulite just melt away. Some of the therapies and ideas outlined in this book may seem strange at first, especially as they are unlikely to be endorsed or recommended by your average doctor.

This book is for all those women who have been made miserable by dimpled bulges on their thighs, bulges they thought they had to put up with for all of their lives. Cellulite, I have proved for myself, is not an unavoidable curse of Eve – it is treatable and removable.

You'll not only feel and look far better without the cellulite deposits, your general health will improve as well. Since I got rid of mine I have found that my energy levels have increased considerably. Walking around with those unnecessary bulges was actually making me more tired than I need be.

All I can say is – there is no comparison between life with cellulite and life without it.

CHAPTER ONE

THE EVIDENCE FOR CELLULITE

Does cellulite really exist?

This has got to be the first question asked, as very many people, including some who have loads of cellulite, will tell you that it does not, and that it is merely a fancy new word for old-fashioned fat.

Cellulite is the popular name given to those peculiarly female bulges which collect on thighs, buttocks and upper arms, and which go into 'orange-peel' puckers when pressed and squeezed. But if you ask the average British or American doctor about cellulite, you will probably be laughed to scorn and told categorically that there is no such thing. Doctors, on the whole, will tell you that fat is fat and that is that. And there is some basis for their insistence that 'cellulite' is just so much nonsense. The word does not appear in any medical dictionary, and the condition is not described in any English language medical textbook. There has not been, so far as I know, a single clinical trial on the subject. There have been no research papers on cellulite at all, no letters to *The Lancet* about it, and no studies published in any respected medical journal. There is a condition called *cellulitis*, which is the inflammation of cellular tissue when a wound turns septic, but this is a serious condition which bears no relation to the cellulite we are talking about.

Cellulite is a French word which has been adopted by alternative practitioners and beauty therapists simply because there is no other word in the English language to describe the kind of lumpy fat deposits which tend to collect on various parts of the female anatomy.

No doctor can, of course, deny the observable fact that very many women have lumps and bumps on their thighs, and that these bulges do present an 'orange-peel' appearance. But are doctors right in believing that the bulges are formed from exactly the same kind of fat as that found everywhere on our bodies? The average doctor in this country will tell you that under the miscroscope, there is no difference between the so-called 'cellulite' areas and other fat cells.

But one should not assume that because the existence of cellulite is denied in orthodox medical circles in Britain and America this holds for the rest of the world. In France, the story is very different. Over there, cellulite has been accepted as a genuine medical condition for the past forty years. So much do they accept its existence that you can have anti-cellulite treatments on their equivalent of the National Health Service. French doctors believe that cellulite is not, strictly speaking, fat at all, but a kind of water retention. They believe the condition is caused by the action of female hormones on water and body wastes, and that it can, if untreated, lead to serious health problems such as arthritis.

British doctors are aware that cellulite is something the French take seriously – which is probably one more reason why British medicine gives it short shrift. As late as June 1988 Professor Sam Shuster, consultant dermatologist at the Royal Victoria Infirmary, Newcastle, was referring to cellulite as 'a French load of old cobblers'. His explanation of cellulite was that women have less collagen – the protein which gives skin its thickness – in their bodies than men, and because of this the lumps and bumps are more likely to show through. Men do have these bumps and bulges, according to Shuster, but because their skin is thicker we just don't see them. Professor Shuster wasn't denying the existence of the lumps and bumps – just denying that they could be a type of fat unique to women.

Eugenia Chandris, author of *The Venus Syndrome*, investigated cellulite when trying to understand the reason for her own extremely bottom-heavy shape. She too came rapidly to the conclusion that it was no different from ordinary fat. She writes: 'The cellulite question is not supported by any sound medical evidence. In fact, most doctors disdainfully deny the existence of cellulite: they say it is just ordinary fat. What is the truth?'

Chandris, who eventually resorted to extremely painful plastic surgery to correct her own Christina Onassis-type 'thunder thighs', felt along with Professor Shuster that the only reason we see the stuff on women is because their skin is finer and the lumps and bumps show through more.

Chandris, of Greek origin like Christina Onassis, had been plagued by jodhpur thighs ever since she was a young teenager. Her mother, fearing that such a shape would ruin her chances of making a good marriage, sent her all over the world to try out patent cures and medicines. Nothing worked and, in the end, she seemed to have no choice but to go for plastic surgery.

Her book was published in 1986, many years after the word 'cellulite' first crossed the Channel and the condition was being treated by alternative practitioners.

So who is right? Is there such a thing as cellulite, a women-only type of fat, or is it just something dreamed up by commercial companies who want to make lots of money out of we foolish women? Are all French doctors really talking a load of old cobblers when they accept the existence of cellulite?

Ten years ago, I was as sceptical as most of the British doctors, thinking it was extremely unlikely that there could be a special type of fat which only women possessed. After all, fat cells were fat cells. It was well known that women were predisposed to the pear shape, whereas men tended to be 'apples' and collect fat round their middles. Women became pear-shaped and men got beer bellies. That was an observable difference between the sexes, and both kinds of fat were, it seemed, caused by a combination of over-indulgence in food and drink and under-indulgence in physical activity. Also, it was a fact that metabolism slowed down as people aged, and that middle-aged spread and middle-aged thighs were part of growing older. It was just that differences in anatomy meant that men's and women's fat tended to collect in different places.

Several explanations were offered by the medical profession as to why this happened. One was that female lower-body fat served a biological purpose. It was there in case of famine, so that women – who had to reproduce the next generation – would have fat stores for themselves and their unborn babies to feed on, if necessary.

Another explanation was that this type of fat was just an extension of 'womanly curves', which had been provided by nature to make women's bodies soft and appealing, as different as possible from the hard, hairy bodies of men.

A third explanation was that it was the result of gravity. As we got older, obesity experts solemnly assured us, it was only natural that fat would tend to collect in the lower body regions. But this theory, while sounding perfectly logical initially, proved after a minute's thought to be so much nonsense. It could not explain why it was only female thighs that were subject to the laws of gravity. Surely these laws could not be so sexist?

In America, cellulite was seen as a natural, if regrettable, aspect of being a woman. In this country too, we were told by people such as romantic novelist Barbara Cartland that we should not attempt to get rid of this fat, as men liked something 'to grab hold of'.

Although I and very many other women had little choice but to accept these theories, there remained at the back of my mind a nagging doubt. Having been assured time and time again that cellulite did not exist I could not quite understand why I should see it so clearly every time I glanced down at my naked thighs. I had been told that this was just ordinary fat, but if so, why did it collect only in certain places? And why was it that no dieting or exercise regimes did anything to diminish the dimples?

It didn't take tremendous powers of observation for me to

see for myself that many women who had cellulite were not otherwise fat. There was, quite clearly, something that was different about it. There had to be some good reason, too, why only women collected bulgy fat on their thighs, and men never did.

However much we were told that cellulite did not exist we still didn't like it being there. So when patent anti-cellulite treatments began appearing on the market in the mid-seventies (most of them hailing from France) we fell for them.

Of course, British doctors lost no time in warning us against these patent cures, saying that there was no evidence whatever that they could work to melt fat away from thighs. The very existence of these creams, concocted, the manufacturers told us, from precious herbal extracts distilled by a mysterious process, seemed to give credence to the medical profession's firmly held conviction that the concept of cellulite had been invented by cosmetic companies to foist yet another unnecessary product onto the ever-gullible consumer. All you had to do, the doctors cynically observed, was to play on female vanity and you had a licence to print money.

These new anti-cellulite creams were beguilingly advertised and presented. The message was that they were specially designed to rid problem areas of ugly lumps and bumps. The products were always illustrated with a picture of a beautiful young woman blessed with the slenderest thighs, the implication being that a diligent application of the cream could give you the same kind of enviable legs.

I wanted to believe the claims made by the manufacturers

of these creams, but common sense seemed to tell me that they couldn't possibly work. It appeared most likely that they belonged in exactly the same category as hair restorers, bust enlargers and pills to restore sexual potency and attractiveness. In other words, they were preying on universal fears ripe for exploitation by the get-rich-quick merchants since the beginning of time.

Of course, the products didn't even begin to work. Those of us who tried them found that however hard we rubbed them in, the lumps and bumps remained as firmly in place as ever. So of course more than ever we seemed to have no choice but to believe the doctors who assured us that cellulite was an invention by those dastardly Frogs, who believed they could foist anything on a naïve and unsuspecting British public.

Before long, the Advertising Standards Authority stepped in to say that the claims made for most of these creams and lotions were unsupported by any scientific evidence and should be withdrawn. As a result, the claims that these products could magically melt away fat, themselves melted away and were replaced by more innocuous wording, such as that they could 'improve circulation'. Well, you couldn't argue about the ability of a cream to improve circulation if you rubbed it in vigorously enough.

Most of these products stayed on the market, however, although sales must have been adversely affected. But the fact that these highly expensive French creams sold at all highlights the despair of millions of women who know they have lumpy, bulging thighs that they hate, whatever the doctors say.

Then, around 1981, came a breakthrough in my own understanding of the problem, enabling me to view cellulite in a completely new way. I was asked by a newspaper to write an article on the subject, pulling together all the latest views and theories. The controversy over whether it did or did not exist had reared up again, for some reason. As expected, all the doctors and obesity experts I consulted reiterated their belief that cellulite was a figment of hysterical women's imagination.

This time I didn't leave it there. I contacted Celia Wright, who with her husband Brian runs a forward-thinking nutrition centre in Sussex. Celia and Brian have both spent many years investigating and trying out all the new theories on nutrition and health, and approach everything completely openmindedly. To them, any theory is innocent until proved guilty.

Celia firmly believed that cellulite did exist and that it was not merely something dreamed up by French cosmetic companies with French franc signs in their eyes. 'As I see it,' she told me, 'cellulite isn't really fat at all in the strict sense of the word. It's actually toxic waste material that the body cannot get rid of in the ordinary way, and has dumped to far-off sites, well out of the way of vital organs.'

She further explained that the reason only women suffer from cellulite is a hormonal one, recognized by French doctors all those years ago. The female hormone oestrogen, said Celia, acts to send toxins to thighs, buttocks and upper arms because it has a protective as well as a reproductive function. Oestrogen works to protect vital organs in case of pregnancy. Men don't get cellulite because there is not the same vital need to protect their bodies from collecting rubbish. Whereas women get cellulite, men get furred-up arteries. (It is actually medically known that oestrogen protects women from coronary heart disease, and that this is why women usually succumb to heart attacks only after the menopause, when oestrogen is no longer circulating.)

I had never heard this explanation before but instantly it began to make sense. If cellulite is, as Celia said, accumulated toxic waste rather than real fat, it would explain why no amount of dieting and exercise would ever shift the stuff. If oestrogen plays an important part in the formation of cellulite, this could be the reason why only women get it.

It would also shed light on male doctors' persistent denial of the existence of cellulite. Of course they often are not particularly interested in female-only problems.

So why is it, I asked Celia Wright, that the body cannot eliminate these so-called toxins? (You have to remember that even in the early 1980s most doctors laughed at the idea that the human body could harbour 'toxins' for years on end. Their view was that the body was perfectly well-equipped with organs of elimination, and that no modern diets were poisonous, anyway.)

Celia explained that in normal circumstances the body's own waste disposal system does an excellent job. The problem is that these days many of us overload our bodies with processed foods, coffee, alcohol, cigarettes, environmental pollution – and in the end, the system simply can't cope. It does its best, but there is sometimes just too much waste for it to handle. The main reason why cellulite stays in place, she added, and is so very difficult to get rid of, is that once the body sends the rubbish to thighs, buttocks and upper arms it reckons it has done its job of waste disposal. So it forgets all about the stuff and makes no further effort to shift it.

After I had heard Celia's theory, I began to read books and articles on the subject by other nutritional experts, such as Leslie Kenton and herbalist Kitty Campion. They were all saying exactly the same things about cellulite – that it wasn't real fat, that it was a waste disposal problem, and that it was caused by eating the wrong kinds of food and living the wrong kind of lifestyle, rather than by simply eating too much and taking too little exercise.

It seemed to me that either these women were just repeating each other's cranky theories, or they knew something that doctors didn't. The difficulty, of course, was that none of them is a qualified doctor – Celia Wright and Leslie Kenton are entirely self-taught, and Kitty Campion has trained as a herbalist, which is a speciality not recognized by conventional doctors.

Alternative practitioners had always maintained that cellulite did exist. But until the alternative medicine revolution of the eighties, these practitioners were held in low esteem by the medical profession. Now, with the interest in the relationship between diet and health and natural therapies, they began to come into their own, and people began to take what they had to say more seriously.

After studying the subject properly and listening to what alternative therapists had to say on the subject I came to the definite conclusion that cellulite exists. The toxic waste explanation made far more sense than any other I had heard, and in addition it accorded perfectly with all the new ideas on health and nutrition which were being increasingly accepted by open-minded people.

By turning myself into my own guinea pig I have proved conclusively to my own satisfaction that cellulite is a different problem from ordinary fat. Whereas once I was plagued with acres of the stuff, now I have none at all. I did not find any scientific or medical papers on the subject, and it was only when I accepted the 'alternative' explanation and tried the 'alternative' treatments that my cellulite began to disappear.

However, even now most British doctors are denying the existence of cellulite. By and large, they have not been persuaded. This is what Dr David Delvin, a well-known media doctor and 'agony uncle' to several women's magazines, has to say about it, writing in the doctors' journal *General Practitioner* in May 1988: 'Many people have great difficulty in losing an excessive bulge from their bottoms. As you probably know, women's magazines and beauty clinics tend to promote the idea that these bulges are extremely hard to shift because they contain a mysterious substance called cellulite.

'Personally, I don't know of any evidence that cellulite actually *exists* – and you certainly won't find it in the pages of Muir's *Pathology* textbook.'

I'm inclined to think that Muir (presumably a man) might learn something if he listened to herbalists, aromatherapists and holistic healers. They are convinced that cellulite does exist, and that it is an eminently treatable condition – without resorting to painful and expensive cosmetic surgery.

In his article, Dr Delvin went on to say that the 'orange-peel' fat can be removed by a horrific-sounding surgical operation which is extremely painful and 'fairly drastic'.

But it's not at all necessary. Once you accept that cellulite is a visible sign that the body is harbouring toxic wastes, you can then embark on treatments which enable the poisons to disperse, rather than using the surgeon's knife to slice it away.

CHAPTER TWO

THE CAUSES OF CELLULITE

I think we can safely assume that cellulite does exist, whatever some doctors may say to the contrary, and that it is a major problem for thousands of women in the world today.

Every woman who has cellulite would rather not have it. But having been assured by countless medical 'experts' that the stuff doesn't exist, the cellulite sufferer has assumed it is just something she has to put up with, just another of the difficulties which go with being a woman.

This is not so. Nature never meant us to have cellulite and we would all be a lot better off without it. But before attempting any successful anti-cellulite regime it is essential to understand exactly what cellulite is, why it develops, and what will make it go away. It becomes possible to get rid of it once you understand why it forms.

So how do you know whether you've got cellulite in the first place? One of the main characteristics is dimples. You know you've got cellulite on your legs if they have a dimply appearance when you stand up. Another factor is that cellulite areas feel cold to the touch. This is because circulation is poor in those areas.

Almost always, the skin on cellulite areas is whiter and more difficult to tan than other skin.

Cellulite is not flab, and it is not fat. Flabby skin does not have the dimpled appearance, and nor does ordinary fat. If you pinch an area containing cellulite you will find that it stays up for far longer than skin pinched, say, on the forearm. This indicates that the fat cells are waterlogged. If it is allowed to accumulate, it becomes hard and grainy. In the early stages it is soft because of the presence of fluid, but becomes progressively harder as the years go by. The harder cellulite is, the more difficult it becomes to lose, although it is never impossible.

The presence of cellulite is nothing to do with being overweight. You can be verging on anorexia and still have cellulite deposits. Conversely, you can be extremely fat and still not have any cellulite on your legs.

If you do have it, though, you should do all you can to get rid of the stuff. For it indicates that your body is in a toxic condition. If the cellulite is left untreated, the toxicity could lead to more serious conditions, such as arthritis or permanent water retention. The presence of cellulite is a warning that your body needs a thorough cleanse and detoxification.

The Discovery of Cellulite

Is cellulite a new problem, brought about by the artificiality of modern living, or has it always existed? Of course, it is difficult to be certain, as the concept and treatment did not come into being until about forty years ago. But, looking at certain Old Master paintings, it seems as though cellulite certainly existed in the seventeenth century. Many of the nudes in Rubens' paintings, for instance, seem to have loads of cellulite. Patricia Davis, who was one of the first British aromatherapists to develop a successful cellulite cure, believes that it is not a new phenomenon at all.

'Most of Rembrandt's nude paintings were of his second wife – and boy, did she have cellulite,' Patricia said. 'All the characteristics are there – the dimpliness, the whiteness, the bulges. The classic painting of a woman with cellulite is the one where she is stepping into water semi-nude, and you just see the texture of her thighs, which are a dead giveaway.

'It seems extremely reasonable to suppose that cellulite existed in Holland in the sixteenth and seventeenth centuries. After all, the Dutch diet was high in dairy produce and the rich women would have led extremely sedentary lives. So I doubt that it's all that new, although few people would have bothered about it much when thighs were never normally exposed.'

Patricia Davis says that she first became aware of cellulite as a medical problem in France around 1952, when she was studying ballet there. 'At that time, the condition was attributed to water retention, and was considered treatable,' she said. 'In fact, we now know that although cellulite and water retention are linked, they are not exactly the same thing.

'The standard treatment in those days was hydrotherapy at one of the famous spas, where extremely fierce jets of water would be applied to the affected areas. Hydrotherapy is the medicinal equivalent to a jacuzzi. The treatment worked, because you got a lot of pummelling, which would drive the cellulite out of the fat cells and help it to disperse. This treatment was backed up by lots of ordinary massage, mud baths and a "nature cure" diet.

'In the 1950s the condition was thought to be caused by poor kidney function, which meant that excess water could not be excreted. Now of course, we know that cellulite is caused by a sluggish lymphatic system. But certainly in France it was always recognized as a woman-only problem.'

Patricia became interested in the question of diet and health when, at the early age of twenty-six, she developed severe arthritis. She gave up dancing when her first child was born, and soon her arthritis was so bad that she could not even walk down the street.

'My doctor told me that I had given up dancing too quickly, and that arthritis was always a danger for dancers and athletes who suddenly stop. I was put on some drugs which were later found to be highly dangerous, but the condition just got worse. In those days – 1956 – nobody ever spoke about curing yourself through diet. It would have been considered extremely cranky.

'But one day a friend said, "Why don't you try the nature cure?" She lent me a book written in the 1930s, and everything I read made complete sense. I put myself straight-away on what we would now call a healthy diet, and cured my own arthritis completely. Since going on the nature cure I have never had even a twinge.

'That opened my eyes to the powerful effect food can have on bodies. Having made myself completely symptom-free I helped other people with arthritis, and then realized I could treat those with chronic illnesses.'

When her children were young Patricia ran a ballet school, but later she trained as an aromatherapist and masseuse and set up business in the mid 1960s. It was then that she began to realize the extent of the cellulite problem. In those days, she said, women did not come to her for their cellulite, as most had no idea they were suffering from any kind of treatable condition. They just assumed that the lumps and bumps were somehow supposed to be there, just the way they were made.

'Very many of my clients were coming to me because of a weight problem,' she said. 'But as I massaged them, I realized that many hadn't got a weight problem at all but were suffering from cellulite instead. I would tell them that it wasn't fat they had, but cellulite, and they would say: but what's that?'

Since there were no textbooks to guide her, Patricia Davis began treating cellulite with hard massage and essential oils. 'It was simply trial and error,' she told me. 'I knew from my aromatherapy training that certain essential oils did help the body to cleanse and detoxify, and that others were stimulating for circulation. The effect of certain essential oils has been very well documented in France, and I simply applied this knowledge to the cellulite problem.

'I knew all about detoxifying diets from treating my own arthritis, and so I just put the two bits of knowledge together. If, as I suspected, cellulite was a toxic condition, then the diet plus massage and aromatherapy treatments would get rid of it. And of course, it did.

'But I have to say that I and other aromatherapists were proceeding very much from theory. In the early days, it was a

27

matter of backing a hunch, as we had no medical textbooks to guide us. It was all very difficult, as our treatments and suggestions were being completely derided by orthodox doctors, who regarded us as charlatans and cranks.'

In many ways, the story of cellulite can be compared to the pre-menstrual tension saga. In the 1920s and 1930s there was no mention whatever of PMT in any medical textbook. So far as the mainly male medical profession was concerned, the condition simply didn't exist. All 'female problems' were just evidence that women were the weaker sex and had to be humoured and pacified like children. And of course, all doctors knew the correct cure for period problems of any kind – go away and have a baby.

It wasn't until gynaecologist Dr Katharina Dalton began to ask pertinent questions about hormonal fluctuations in women that the syndrome began to be recognized, named, and written up in medical literature. This was in 1953. When Dr Dalton began training as a doctor she was already married with three children, and had noticed that whenever she became pregnant the headaches, depression, heaviness and bloating that she suffered from just before a period, went away. Of course, in those days, the term 'pre-menstrual tension' had not been invented. But through study and research, Dr Dalton came to realize that it was a medical condition suffered by very many women, and that it was treatable.

Now, of course, her conclusions are accepted by all doctors, several of which have set up special PMT clinics. PMT is big business nowadays, and huge sums of money are being made out of patent treatments such as evening primrose oil and vitamin B6. Consequently it is hard to realize that only forty years ago doctors were assuring women there was no such thing as PMT. Problems associated with menstruation were, like many women-only complaints, seen as trivial.

Over the past few years there has been much research on PMT. Since about 1980 it has been established that there is a definite connection between PMT and the lack of certain vitamins, minerals and essential fatty acids. This explosion of knowledge on the subject means that there is no longer any reason for women to suffer from PMT – at least, not in silence.

The same thing now needs to happen with cellulite. Unlike PMT, which comes and goes, cellulite is an ever-present problem. There is plenty of evidence to suggest that it is caused by the wrong kind of diet, stress, prescription drugs, a sedentary lifestyle, too much tea, coffee and alcohol, cigarettes, poor circulation and a sluggish lymphatic system.

Although cellulite has probably always existed, it seems reasonable to suppose that the problem is getting worse. The main reason for this is that more women than ever now smoke, drink, eat processed foods and take prescription drugs, such as the pill. All of these alter hormonal balance and may well affect the workings of vital organs.

The other factor which has a bearing on our new awareness of cellulite is that it is only in the latter half of this century that women generally began exposing their legs and thighs. In the past, that was confined to artists' models. In the mid-1960s, with the advent of miniskirts, the standard explanation of bulgy thighs was that they were caused by cold weather. If girls were daft enough to walk around in the middle of winter with skirts halfway up their thighs they must expect some bulges, doctors seriously said.

They then explained cellulite by saying that the body developed extra layers of fat to cope with the cold. For a time, we all believed this. But then when miniskirts went out of fashion to be replaced by midi skirts and the bulges still didn't go away, that theory fell into disuse.

To me, the most telling evidence for the existence of cellulite is the neat appearance of French women over 'a certain age'. Whereas the majority of middle-aged English women have thighs absolutely thick with cellulite, it is noticeably absent from the legs of French ladies. Now, either French women are constructed completely differently from their English counterparts, or they have learned something that we still need to learn – that cellulite is a problem which can be treated.

Not that cellulite is a problem confined to older women by any means. The condition can appear as early as the age of twelve or thirteen and then remain for life, unless treated.

How Do We Get Cellulite, and Why?

Cellulite is a problem confined to women. Men never get it. As such, it is safe to assume that there is a hormonal factor involved. In fact. it seems most likely – and I have to say 'seems' because there are no proper medical studies on the subject – that the condition is caused, above all, by the presence of oestrogen. The more oestrogen there is in a woman's body, the more likely it is that cellulite will develop. The danger times for developing cellulite are at puberty, pregnancy and the menopause, the times of greatest hormonal fluctuation.

Cellulite was first thought to have a hormonal component when French doctors realized that men never suffered from it. It was then discovered that the female hormone oestrogen predisposes women towards retaining fluid. From there, it was a short step towards an understanding that oestrogen must somehow be implicated in the formation of cellulite.

Unless women are frequently pregnant, they have high levels of oestrogen circulating around their system continuously. The amount of oestrogen circulating in women's bodies has also increased enormously since the mid 1960s with the introduction of the contraceptive pill and hormone replacement therapy for post-menopausal women.

Oestrogen has a specific purpose, and that is to prepare the body to receive and nurture an embryo. Whenever pregnancy occurs, the amount of oestrogen circulating in the system drops rapidly. Nowadays most women have far more oestrogen circulating in their system than was intended by nature. It acts to send waste materials away from vital organs and into areas where they will be relatively harmless. This eventually becomes apparent as cellulite. In men, waste products have the effect of furring up their arteries, so they are more likely to succumb to heart attacks. It seems as if biology acts to protect the female. We get cellulite, whereas men get hardening of the arteries – a condition which is taken extremely seriously by most doctors. What they have not realized yet is that cellulite and coronary heart disease are different manifestations of an identical problem – too much stress, a bad diet, too little exercise, and too much rubbish getting into the system and not being able to get out.

Although men don't have cellulite some of them do have beer bellies, which are a related problem caused mainly by the high oestrogen content of hops. It is also noticeable that men who are very heavy beer drinkers often suffer from female-type breast development. This is yet another indication that oestrogen appears to predispose towards the retention of unwanted fluid.

Recent studies on the contraceptive pill have linked it with the formation of breast cancer and an increased incidence of thrombosis. Dr Ellen Grant, an early researcher into oral contraception and now one of the pill's most outspoken opponents, believes that it is linked with general bad health in women. She argues that the pill significantly interferes with carbohydrate metabolism and blood function. Studies carried out by Professor Victor Wynn at the metabolic unit, St Mary's Hospital, in London, have shown that the pill encourages blood fats to increase. It also stops the uptake of certain essential minerals such as zinc, iron and magnesium, and encourages an excess of copper to stay in the system.

Dr Grant does not mention in her book *The Bitter Pill* that oral contraception encourages the formation of cellulite, but from what we know about the action of oestrogen it seems extremely likely that this is so. Although cellulite is very probably not a new problem, as far as we can tell it appears to be far more prevalent in the late twentieth century than at any other time in history.

The contraceptive pill is, of course, formulated from

synthetic hormones. But the body does not distinguish between synthetic and natural hormones, and so far as the female system is concerned, taking the pill simply means that the oestrogen action on the body is increased.

Ellen Grant believes that oral contraceptives interfere with body metabolism and the release of complex biochemical substances. They can also cause far-reaching blood and circulatory changes and can lead to weight gain and breast tenderness.

Another factor, most probably linked to hormones, is that women's bodies simply cannot take the same amount of punishment and abuse that men's can. We know now for a fact that women's tolerance threshold for alcohol and nicotine is far lower than men's. But all the time women are abusing their bodies, oestrogen performs its powerful protective function, and does its best to send the waste to outlying areas so that we will survive.

The reason most of us don't feel ill when we have a cellulite problem is that the body has been successful in sending the rubbish far away from vital organs. With men, the rubbish is retained nearer the centre, which is why they are far more likely to suffer from heart, circulatory and blood pressure problems.

To sum up, we can say that cellulite forms when there is a general circulatory problem in the body. It is, above all, an indication of a sluggish circulation, a sign that body wastes cannot be disposed of in the normal way. When cellulite is present, this means that the lymphatic system, the body's main vacuum cleaner, cannot do its job, and that there is internal clogging.

The next step is to understand exactly what causes the clogging in the first place. Because once this is understood, we can set about unclogging the system.

The Main Causes of Cellulite

There is very little we can do to decrease the amount of oestrogen circulating in our bodies. But oestrogen will not send rubbish to outlying areas unless there is rubbish to send. So the first thing to understand about cellulite is that it is caused mainly by leading the wrong lifestyle. The body is very clever at recognizing the difference between nutrients and anti-nutrients, and does all it can to neutralize the effect of those substances which it does not need, and which actually have a harmful effect.

COFFEE
Of all cellulite-causing substances, probably the most harmful is coffee, because of the caffeine it contains. The bad effects of coffee have now been well documented, and several medical studies have suggested that more than three cups a day can do damage. None of the studies mentions cellulite, of course, as a possible adverse side-effect of caffeine, but the substance has now been definitely linked with all kinds of female complaints from benign breast lumps to pelvic disorders. Caffeine interferes with the uptake of certain essential minerals in the diet, particularly iron, and also predisposes to certain anxiety states.

The main reason for this is that caffeine puts extra stress on the adrenal glands, which release adrenalin. Like cocaine, caffeine gives the system an instant boost by making the adrenals pump out extra adrenalin. The problem is that when we drink huge amounts of coffee, we enable large quantities of adrenalin to be released which are not burned up at all. Biologically, adrenalin exists to protect us from danger, to enable us to run away or to stay and fight. We naturally get surges of adrenalin when there is a near miss on the motorway, when we are about to take an important exam or attend a vital interview. Then, when the danger is past, the adrenalin production ceases. Caffeine enables this hormone to be secreted all the time.

So coffee puts extra stress on the adrenals by overworking them. They discharge too much adrenalin into the system and become exhausted. Too much caffeine in the system also puts extra stress onto the kidneys, where all water-soluble rubbish is taken so that the blood can be cleansed.

It is now well known that a high intake of caffeine puts people at extra risk of heart attack, as it increases the amount of cholesterol in the system. This causes even more clogging up. In women, the net result of overconsumption is to increase the amount of cellulite on the thighs. For most women, the presence of cellulite is a potent indicator that they are drinking too much caffeine, in the form of tea, coffee, or colas. Chocolate also contains a significant amount of caffeine.

Drinks containing caffeine make you feel good by giving you an instant lift, but this is followed not much later by a nasty low – the well-known withdrawal symptoms. In women who are pregnant or on the pill, caffeine is eliminated particularly slowly, which indicates a hormonal link.

Furthermore, coffee beans are loaded with pesticides, which in large quantities can upset the digestive process. There is no particular advantage in drinking tea, either, as it also contains significant amounts of caffeine, though only half as much as coffee and, in addition, can be loaded with impurities such as copper. Consuming anti-nutrients means that the deposits of cellulite can only get bigger.

In the past, both women and men would have drunk very little coffee. It was first introduced into the Western world in the eighteenth century, and for a long time was confined to men drinking it occasionally in the famous coffee houses. It was not until the 1920s that women began to drink coffee every day, and the development of instant coffee – even worse for you than the filtered variety – meant that we could all drink vast amounts every day.

Now, of course, coffee is the favourite non-alcoholic beverage among young women. Very many women also drink vast quantities of tea, thinking nothing of downing five or six cups a day.

Possibly one of the reasons the French recognized cellulite so long ago was that they have for a long time been a nation of dedicated coffee-drinkers. Coffee and tea have now become our most universal stimulants, and we tend to forget that, delicious though they may be, they are actually non-nutrients, substances the body emphatically does not need for its daily functioning.

The potentially addictive quality of tea and coffee is a warning sign, or should be. The body develops specific cravings only when its biochemistry has been artificially adapted to accommodate an alien substance. If you give your body just what it needs for proper functioning, cravings and addictions do not develop. Unfortunately, in our present society, we have mistaken cravings and addictions for excitement. We appear to thrive on artificial sensual stimulation, forgetting that the human body was not originally designed to cope with these substances. It is hardly surprising if, after a time, it cannot cope with the onslaught and starts to rebel.

Of course, not everybody who consumes vast quantities of caffeine will get cellulite any more than every single person who smokes will die of lung cancer. Some systems can withstand large amounts of stimulating beverages, others can't. The fact is, though, that caffeine significantly adds to the burden on the body.

NICOTINE

Nicotine, like caffeine, is extremely bad for women. It is bad for men as well, but it seems that woman's system is less able to withstand the poisons released by tobacco in the bloodstream. We have known for twenty years or more that smoking during pregnancy causes low-birthweight babies and, more recently, it has also been linked with malformations and brain damage in embryos.

The first effect of nicotine is that it uses up oxygen, reducing the amount available for use by the cells. It does this by decreasing the efficiency of the lungs. It also affects the haemoglobin – red cells – in the blood. Haemoglobin is the main carrier for oxygen in the blood, and picks up the oxygen in the lungs as the blood circulates.

If the oxygen exchange in the blood is less efficient because of nicotine intake, then every cell in the body will receive less oxygen than it should. This factor is extremely relevant to the cellulite problem because, above all, oxygen acts as a powerful stimulator and cleanser for the blood. Body cells cannot function without adequate oxygen any more than we can ourselves. Whenever there is reduced oxygen in the body, cell function is impaired and circulation is adversely affected.

Some anti-cellulite therapists in America are now noticing that the problem is worse in young girls than in middle-aged women. The main reason for this, they theorize, is increased cigarette consumption. Because although older women – and men – are now significantly reducing their nicotine intake, the habit is becoming more prevalent among young people.

A recent large-scale study among schoolchildren in Britain revealed that teenage girls are now smoking far more than teenage boys. In addition, they find it more difficult to give up, and are more likely to become addicted smokers by the time they are in their mid-twenties. The main reasons given for taking up the habit were release of tension, and a desire to appear sophisticated, 'cool' and grown up.

Smoking adds to the amount of toxic wastes that enter the body, which means that the system has to work even harder to get rid of them. Nicotine is a powerful pollutant and, like caffeine, it is an anti-nutrient. Its effect is to rob the system of essential substances such as Vitamin C and zinc.

A report by the Royal College of Physicians in 1983 provides some useful figures on women and smoking. Few women, according to the report, smoked before the Second World War but by 1956 around forty-two per cent of women in Britain aged sixteen and over were smokers. Since that time, there has been a steady decline, with around thirty-seven per cent of British women smoking today. The vast majority of these are women under the age of twenty-five.

It has been known for decades that women who smoke are at vastly increased risk from heart disease and all diseases of the circulatory system. It has also now been established that smoking affects fertility and results in an earlier menopause.

The Royal College's report states that women seem to find it harder than men to give up smoking, and adds that the reason for this is unclear. One major reason why women continue to smoke is that they are are afraid of gaining weight if they give up. Smoking increases metabolism, and also provides an alternative to eating when some kind of comfort is needed. But as smoking affects circulation, it also adds to cellulite deposits which are, of course, as much a problem as overweight.

The anti-cellulite programme outlined in this book ensures that smoking can be given up without any danger at all of unwelcome weight gain.

ALCOHOL

As with cigarettes and coffee, alcohol consumption was not a significant factor for women until the 1920s, the so-called 'flapper age' when cocktails became popular and it was suddenly fashionable for women to drink. Nowadays, most women drink alcohol regularly.

Women can take far less alcohol than men. One reason for

this is that female livers are smaller and able to process less. Another reason is that women's bodies have a higher proportion of fat than men's, and alcohol does not enter fat cells. This means that its effect is concentrated into a smaller area and takes longer to be processed by the liver.

Alcohol enters the blood very quickly and instantly alters blood chemistry. It adds to the workload of the liver, which can then very quickly become overloaded. When alcohol is added to the sum total of non-nutrients entering the body the result is that the liver and kidneys cannot effectively handle the excess waste material. For most people, the eliminative organs have enough to do handling ordinary waste materials produced by the diet. If they have to deal with caffeine, nicotine and alcohol loads as well it is not surprising that they find it hard to cope, and that much waste matter simply stays in the system.

DIET

Although deposits of cellulite can be seen clearly in the paintings of Rubens, Rembrandt and Renoir, it is unlikely that women living in pre-literate societies ever collected much of the stuff. In fact, very few women living what we might call a 'natural' life – eating wholefoods, lots of fruit and vegetables and not drinking tea, coffee or alcohol – ever develop a cellulite problem.

In the modern West, the eliminative difficulties caused by smoking, coffee and alcohol consumption are exacerbated by an artificial diet. In recent years we have of course been urged to eat more fruit and vegetables, brown rice and wholemeal bread in order to stave off serious diseases. Nutritionists say that we were designed to eat a pure, wholefood diet and to experience stress only at certain times, such as when specific dangers threatened. We have already seen how a high caffeine intake adds to the number of stress hormones circulating round the body. Excess stress is also placed on body systems by eating artificial and processed foods, substances which, like caffeine and alcohol, the body was not designed to cope with.

When a pure, natural diet is eaten, the liver and large intestine are extremely efficient at getting rid of wastes very quickly. In fact, the more natural the food, the quicker the digestive system breaks it down. The more artificial it becomes, the longer it takes to go through the body. In some cases, the artificial substance may not be eliminated by the body at all, and may simply stay in the system, sometimes for years on end. Recent work in America on colon cleansing – which is very similar to the anti-cellulite programme – revealed that years of eating artificial foods mean that waste products are never eliminated from the colon but remain there for ever. Autopsies nowadays often reveal many pounds of waste material which would have been completely eliminated if the system had been working effectively.

Much of the waste material that is not handled by the liver or large intestine gets reabsorbed back into the body, where it starts to do damage. It is when too much waste material accumulates that we notice cellulite deposits. The more the system is clogged up and the more sluggish the circulation becomes, the worse the cellulite problem is likely to be.

Cellulite-encouraging foodstuffs are sugar, dairy produce,

meat and anything processed, smoked or preserved. Sugar has a similar effect on the body to caffeine, in that it releases adrenalin and gives a quick energy boost, followed by a 'down' not long after. Dairy produce is mucus-forming, which means that it encourages waste material to become sticky and stay in the system. Meat products also take a long time to be processed by the body and, in some cases, may never be entirely eliminated.

A SEDENTARY LIFESTYLE
Women who are very active, eat a wholefood diet and abstain from alcohol, cigarettes and caffeine, will rarely get cellulite. These days, very many women have jobs that necessitate sitting at a desk all day long. Prolonged inactivity of this kind can cut off circulation. When treating cellulite, therapists often notice that cellulite deposits are at their most intract-able where the legs meet the chair edge – at the place where circulation is cut off most.

Prolonged physical inactivity leads to an increasingly sluggish circulation, making it even harder for the blood and lymphatic system to get rid of waste materials and send life-giving oxygen round the system.

How Cellulite Forms

Cellulite is, above all, a signal that the body's circulation is slowing down and becoming ineffective. Research carried out in Italy shows clearly that cellulite cells are different from other fat cells. Definite physical changes take place in the cells resulting in enlarged capillaries and a weakening of the capillary walls.

The diagrams (a) and (b) show what happens when fat cells are invaded by cellulite. Diagram (a) shows normal, cellulite-free fat cells, with thin capillaries. Diagram (b) shows the effects of cellulite. The capillaries have become greatly enlarged, and blood plasma has seeped out of them into the surrounding fatty tissue. This causes the fat cells to bunch up together, rather than being widely separated as in the first diagram. The effect of this is that the lymph nodes, which normally would drain away excess fluid, become unable to cope, and so the excess plasma stays in the cells.

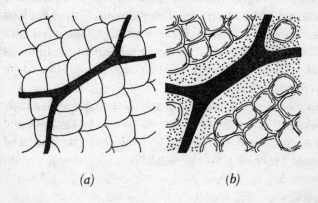

(a)   *(b)*

At the same time as all this is happening, the walls of the fat cells change their structure, to become thickened by extra deposits of collagen. When this takes place, there is further congestion of the circulation, resulting in even more cellulite. So, whenever you have some cellulite, conditions are always created for more to form. The fatty cells become waterlogged and toxin-loaded, full of junk the body simply cannot eliminate.

Cellulite forms when women's bodies produce or take in too much oestrogen, resulting in waste matter being pushed away from vital organs. At the same time as this increased oestrogen pushes the waste away, we are taking in too much junk in the form of food residues, chemicals, artificial additives and preservatives, nicotine, alcohol and tobacco.

As the body was not designed to cope with all these non-nutrients it simply does not know what to do with them. Although the liver can detoxify a certain amount of hormones out of the blood, and keep the bloodstream relatively clear, it cannot manage vastly increased amounts of oestrogen. Nor can it cope with the daily onslaught of junk foods and junk substances. There is no biological mechanism to rid our bodies of the huge amount of junk and pollution which daily invade them.

There are basically two kinds of junk the body has to deal with – the water-soluble kind and the fat-soluble kind. The kidneys handle the former, and the liver looks after the latter. If all the waste material which enters our bodies had to be coped with by the liver we would become seriously ill with liver-related problems. As it is, women are protected by the mechanisms that send the rubbish to out-of-the-way places.

This is the main reason why, although we speak of cellulite 'sufferers', very few of them are ever conscious of the process. They cannot feel the cellulite being formed but are very aware of the unsightly bumps once they have appeared – and they will certainly experience pain when undergoing the kind of hard massage needed to get rid of intractable deposits.

But usually cellulite sufferers feel just the same as any other women. This is because our hormonal structure has acted to protect us in a way that it does not protect men. Patricia Davis says: 'The formation of cellulite is really nature protecting those who have to reproduce the species. A lot of poisons get locked in fatty cells, but this is far better for the system than that they should be trapped in the liver, kidneys or arteries.' She defines cellulite as 'a state in which the cells of the subcutaneous fatty layer are invaded by watery deposits carrying toxic waste matter . . . Poor circulation of the blood and a sluggish lymphatic system underlie this condition, and women who have a sedentary job or lifestyle and take little or no exercise are those most often affected.'

The other factor, says Davis, is a diet high in toxic substances – tea, coffee and alcohol, red meats, animal fats and foods containing additives such as artificial colours, flavourings, preservatives or emulsifying chemicals. Smoking is another toxic risk, and living or working in an atmosphere laden with other people's smoke can be almost as bad.

'When a high level of toxins in the body is found jointly with a poor circulation,' she adds, 'the conditions exist in which cellulite can develop. Circulation becomes sluggish in the affected areas, so not enough life-giving oxygen can reach the cells from the blood. At the same time, toxins lodge in the cells because the flow of blood is not sufficient to carry them away. The lymphatic system becomes overworked and cannot drain the cell fluid away effectively. And so, gradually, the whole area becomes stagnant.'

I don't need any further proof to tell me that cellulite exists. Do you?

I believe that the main reason doctors continue to deny the existence of cellulite is that they have no treatments at all to deal with it. There are no pills which will send it away, and diuretics, which are often prescribed to people with a water-retention problem, can result in serious losses of the essential mineral potassium. Nor will plastic surgery or the newer liposuction successfully eliminate cellulite deposits. Although surgery can be a very effective means of slicing away fat – if you can stand the pain, the expense and the possible complications afterwards – it does not ensure that none will ever return. In fact, if you have a toxic system, the cellulite will come back almost immediately, as you have not solved the problem. You may have cleared the drain for the time being, but you have not tackled the reason for its becoming blocked in the first place.

The anti-cellulite programme outlined in this book is not a treatment worked out by medical doctors. It has been developed over the years by nutritionists, aromatherapists and masseurs – and it is guaranteed to work.

There are no adverse side effects, no harsh drugs to take, and no dangers. If you have cellulite – and it is easy to check this by simple observation and pinching the thighs – then you owe it to yourself to get rid of it as quickly as possible.

After all, who wants a junk-laden system?

CHAPTER THREE

THE ANTI-CELLULITE
PROGRAMME

Although cellulite has been regarded as a medical condition in France for many decades it was not until the early 1980s that a fully successful anti-cellulite regime began to be developed, and used in other countries to help women rid themselves of unwanted and unattractive lumps and bumps.

As there were no clinical trials and no proper studies available on cellulite, the treatments were developed gradually, and by 'alternative' practitioners and therapists rather than doctors. As cellulite began to be understood it was realized that it would not go away permanently until the whole system could be cleaned both inside and out. Because although French doctors had been treating cellulite for many years, they did not understand what made it appear in the first place. They could offer treatment, but not prevention. Now it is possible to offer both.

The first alternative practitioners to provide a successful treatment for cellulite were aromatherapists, who used plant substances known as essential oils to help cleanse and detoxify the system. It was also realized that particular kinds of massage could help disperse lumps and bumps from problem areas.

However, it was not until a detoxifying diet was formulated that a completely successful anti-cellulite 'package' could be put together. The combination of the right diet, massage and the correct essential oils, means that cellulite can be completely eradicated, and the lumpy pockets of fat will disappear for ever.

The modern cellulite cure consists of four main elements: **Diet, Dry Skin Brushing, Aromatherapy and Massage**. All these four ingredients are absolutely essential in any effective anti-cellulite programme, but most vital is the diet. Because, even if you manage to get rid of some cellulite with oils and massage, it will always come back unless you can prevent more forming with the correct diet. The anti-cellulite diet does two main jobs: it cleanses and detoxifies the whole system to enable toxic wastes to be eliminated, and it prevents more cellulite from forming in the future.

The Diet

When embarking on an anti-cellulite regime, it is essential to cleanse and detoxify the system from inside first. So you must begin with a very strict detoxifying diet.

The anti-cellulite diet now used by most therapists and masseurs grew out of research undertaken mainly in America, where it became apparent that very many of our modern illnesses were caused by large amounts of waste matter remaining in the body. Several American doctors began developing diets that could help people with a wide variety of serious illnesses, such as cancer, schizophrenia, arthritis, allergies and heart disease. One of the first of these doctors was Max Gerson, who successfully cured many patients of cancer with his raw-food diet. Then doctors Nathan Pritikin and Carl Pfeiffer began treating heart patients and the mentally ill with diet and nutritional therapies instead of the surgical and drug treatments which had become standard.

Gradually, further studies and research showed that many of our modern illnesses were caused by eating the wrong kinds of foods which eventually set up serious imbalances in the body. Avant-garde doctors in America also began to realize that much illness was caused by faulty elimination and by waste material staying in the system perhaps for years on end. Once the system is clogged up, they argued, the best method of treatment is to unclog it naturally, rather than rely on harsh drugs and purgatives.

These doctors understood that diuretics and laxatives could not be the answer, because as soon as you stopped taking the tablets the original problem would return and the body would start to clog up once more. In any case, many of the drugs had adverse side effects and would not lead to lasting health.

It seemed that what was needed above all was a diet which would help the body to eliminate its own long-held waste matter and encourage the lymphatic system, which transports wastes to eliminative organs, to do its job properly.

The theory was that a natural, wholefood diet would gradually enable the body to rid itself of accumulated undigested rubbish through the liver, kidneys, colon and skin.

It had been well known for several years that one of the reasons for faulty elimination of wastes was that certain foods tended to stay for too long in the system. If foods are not eliminated quickly then they tend to putrefy long before being expelled through the colon. Foods which would aid elimination, therefore, were those which had a quick 'transit time' – that is, they would pass through the entire alimentary tract before they had time to start decomposing.

And the foods which had the quickest transit times were those closest to nature – raw fruits and vegetables. Also, it was found that the quicker the transit time, the better the digestion, and the greater the likelihood of all the nutrients being absorbed.

Food tends to putrefy inside the body just as quickly as it does when left outside the fridge. If you leave fruit and vegetables outside the fridge it is usually several days before they start to go off. Milk left outside the fridge goes off extremely quickly, and meat will start to spoil in less than a day. Exactly the same thing happens inside the body. As the temperature inside the body is around 98.4°F, putrefaction of food takes place far more quickly than at normal room temperature.

The fresher and more natural the food, the more likely it is that it will pass through the body without undergoing any putrefaction whatever. One of the original formulators of the detoxifying diet, American doctor Robert Gray, found that when he ate a hundred per cent raw-food diet his stools lost all of their putrefactive odour and began to smell of whatever fruit he had been eating.

He also came to realize, by studying autopsies, that milk and dairy produce slowed down transit time by forming mucus, a sticky substance which could stick to the walls of the digestive tract and hinder transit time. Dr Gray, and other nutritional experts in America such as Dr Carl Pfeiffer and Nathan Pritikin, began to develop a diet which would help the whole body to cleanse and detoxify itself. This diet consisted mainly of fresh fruits and vegetables, eaten raw whenever possible, and a certain amount of fibre to aid digestion and effective elimination.

Dr Robert Gray was interested above all in cleaning the colon, and developed a diet which would enable accumulated waste matter to be eliminated. He understood that genuine health is impossible if the colon is impacted with old waste material it can no longer get rid of. His book, *The Colon Health Handbook*, explains how colons gradually become more and more impacted with waste material, mainly because we eat foods which encourage rubbish to stay in the system rather than being properly eliminated. In pre-literate societies, where only natural foods are eaten, many diseases associated with modern living simply do not exist.

Dr Gray realized that one of the most important aspects of a clean system is to have a properly working lymphatic system. There are two types of fluid designed to carry body wastes away – the lymph and the blood. Lymph is similar to blood except that it contains no red blood cells. Lymph vessels are contained in every cell in the body, and their job is to collect waste matter and eventually empty it back into the blood stream. The lymph vessels contain one-way valves and are composed of muscle tissue which pumps the lymph through these valves. When it is all working properly, wastes are taken away automatically via this system. When the lymph vessels are sluggish, however, wastes stay and accumulate in body cells. This is basically what happens when cellulite collects.

In its normal state, lymph is a colourless, watery fluid. Whenever there is over-accumulation of sticky mucoid matter, the lymphatic system is unable to remove it, and the result is congestion. So the very first step in getting rid of waste matter which has accumulated in body cells is to cleanse the lymphatic system, and allow excess toxic and mucoid material to drain away.

The best way to cleanse the lymphatic system is to go on a diet which excludes, as far as possible, foods which form mucus and clog up the body cells. Mucus-forming foods are basically dairy produce and fatty meats. Good lymph-clearing foods are fresh fruit and vegetables, organic if possible, wholegrains such as brown rice and millet, wheat-bran and oatbran, lots of mineral water and only the occasional fish, eggs and lean meat. You should also avoid as far as possible alcohol, coffee, tea and cigarettes, substituting them with herb teas and fruit juices.

When therapists offering anti-cellulite treatments read Dr Gray's *The Colon Health Handbook* they instantly applied the principles to the cellulite problem. Clogged-up colons and waterlogged fatty cells are both manifestations of a related problem: failure to eliminate waste material.

The anti-cellulite diet is not a slimming diet in the usual sense. Although you will very probably lose weight while on it that is not its main purpose. The diet is not designed to get rid of ordinary fat so much as to encourage long-held body wastes to disperse. It helps to regard the anti-cellulite eating regime as, above all, a potent method of cleansing the system. The anti-cellulite diet is described in detail in the following chapter but, briefly, it consists of eating only fresh, natural foods and proteins. Normally on an anti-cellulite programme you will be asked to follow a fruit-and-mineral-water-only diet for a few days, to abstain from coffee, alcohol and tea, and to eat no meat or processed foods. After a week or so, the diet can be modified to some extent, but it is important to follow it fairly rigidly if you really want to be free of cellulite.

Dry Skin Brushing

This is also extremely important, as it further helps clearing and cleansing of the lymphatic system. Dry skin brushing is probably an ancient technique, but it was revived in America in the early 1980s when colon-cleansing became all the rage. According to Dr Robert Gray, who recommended body brushing as well as a pure, natural diet for ensuring colon health, skin brushing is a 'highly effective technique for stimulating the expulsion of fresh mucoid material, hardened particulates or impacted mucoid matter, and other obstructions of the lymphatic system. Like the colon, the lymphatic system can contain stagnant accumulations of old waste matter.'

According to Robert Gray, you know when skin brushing is effective because you will begin to see lymph mucoid in the stools.

You have to use the right kind of brush. An ordinary loofah

or bath mitt won't do, nor will those patent self-massagers advertised at high prices. There is only one kind of brush which does an effective job of helping to cleanse the lymphatic system, and that is a long-handled wooden brush made from natural fibres. At first, this kind of brushing will feel strange and unnatural but most people find that they enjoy it once they have become used to the sensation.

You have to begin body brushing at the same time as starting the diet. The two together will work wonders to get rid of cellulite that has been long held in body cells, and will encourage it to disperse. But as cellulite is often very hard to get rid of you may well need the help of aromatherapy and massage as well.

Aromatherapy

Most aromatherapists now offer anti-cellulite treatments. The essential oils used in aromatherapy work in conjunction with the diet and the body brushing to enable waste matter to empty itself into the lymphatic system.

Recent research on essential oils has established that many have a definite therapeutic effect, and that they do make a difference. For many years, aromatherapy was regarded as a 'French load of old cobblers' in much the same way as cellulite itself was (and still is in many circles), but it is rapidly becoming one of the most popular of all complementary therapies. One of the reasons for this is that people are now learning for themselves that it works.

Research carried out by Professor George Dodd of Warwick University has shown that aromatherapy oils are not just nice scents but can be very potent remedies for a wide variety of ailments. There are specific oils for cleansing, detoxifying and stimulating circulation, and all of these will be used by a qualified aromatherapist to help bring about the body changes which will lead to loss of cellulite.

The use of aromatherapy oils to banish cellulite is explained fully in chapter six.

Massage

This is also extremely important. Like aromatherapy, massage was for many years regarded as simply a beauty treatment indulged in by the idle rich. It has also had a rather unfortunate association with sleazy sex parlours. Now it is known that the right kind of massage can have a dramatic effect on the body. The type most often used in anti-cellulite treatments is known as **lymphatic drainage massage**. This is a very hard, tough kind of massage which pummels and kneads away at the cellulite deposits at the same time as activating the lymph nodes.

If you go for professional anti-cellulite treatments you will find that aromatherapy and massage are always used in conjunction with each other.

Exercise

This is an optional extra in any cellulite-banishing regime. Exercise can be very effective once you have managed to get rid of the worst of the cellulite and need to tone up the muscles. But there is not much point in embarking on rigorous exercise programmes while you have large areas of cellulite on your thighs. Although the condition is partly caused by a sedentary lifestyle, vigorous exercise will not make the slightest bit of difference to cellulite deposits that are already there.

In fact, many forms of exercise could make it worse, particularly anything that includes jumping up and down or pounding, such as jogging, jazz dancing, aerobics or California stretch-type exercises. These are emphatically NOT recommended for cellulite removal. They tend to put extra pressure on the joints and encourage the cellulite to harden and become even more impacted.

The best type of exercise is that which is both gentle and brisk at the same time, such as walking or swimming. Swimming is, in fact, excellent for cellulite sufferers as it exercises the legs without putting any undue strain on the joints.

Very often, women who have been on a rigorous anti-cellulite programme find that their legs become flabby and lacking in tone. This is often a temporary condition and can be likened to when you have just had a baby. The minute the baby is born, your stomach is flabby and stretched, like an empty sack. But after a very few weeks it tightens back up again and becomes flat, especially if you do the right kind of exercises to help yourself get back into shape.

Exactly the same process happens with cellulite removal. If the cellulite has been there for a very long time it will leave a certain amount of flab when it finally goes. Because once cellulite starts to disperse everything can happen very quickly – far too quickly for the skin to stay tight. Before long, though, the skin will start to 'fit' of its own accord. The time to embark on exercise is once the worst of the cellulite has gone.

Relaxation and Deep Breathing

Like most nasty things in life, cellulite is made worse by high levels of stress and anxiety, which release extra adrenalin into the system and make the liver work extra hard to try and get rid of the excess.

You should practise deep breathing whenever you have the opportunity, such as when relaxing in the bath. You do it like this: put both hands on your stomach and as you breathe in, inflate the abdomen. Breathe out slowly, letting the abdomen go back in. Repeat this whenever you think of it. This helps more oxygen to get into the system, and improves circulation.

Can I Get Rid of Cellulite by Myself?

The answer to this is yes.

When I decided that I would try and get rid of my own cellulite I immediately booked up several treatments with a therapist who had been trained in lymphatic drainage massage as well as aromatherapy. I decided to enlist the help of a professional because I wanted to see for myself whether the treatments would work, and I was unsure that I would have the motivation all by myself. But it is perfectly possible to rid yourself of cellulite with the complete self-help programme which is outlined in this book.

The advantages of going to a therapist are that you have an objective assessment of your cellulite and your progress is monitored regularly. There is less chance that you will backslide and start drinking huge amounts of coffee or alcohol, or stuff yourself with cream cakes. Also, you can be sure that the right kind of oils will be used and the correct type of massage employed.

The decision whether to book up professional treatments or do it yourself depends on several factors – your pocket, your levels of self-motivation, the availability of trained therapists and the extent of your cellulite.

If you are young – still in your twenties – and have not therefore been a cellulite sufferer for very long, it is relatively easy to get rid of it by yourself. If, though, you are older, and have large amounts of cellulite which have been there for many years, you may find that professional help is invaluable.

When booking up a therapist it is vital that you go to

somebody who really knows what she is doing. Unfortunately, as with all branches of alternative medicine, there is nothing to stop anybody setting up as an aromatherapist and charging high prices for doing precisely nothing. Names and addresses of reputable organizations are given on p. 131.

Those who are not certain whether or not they have cellulite, or whether their problem is simply one of overweight, might find it useful to check with a trained therapist first. A good practitioner will give an honest answer. Do not assume that because you are overweight or have thick thighs that you necessarily have cellulite. Your thick thighs may be simply a genetic inheritance. It's the lumpiness which indicates cellulite deposits, rather than actual girth. Cellulite has a distinctive appearance and must not be confused with ordinary flab or muscle. The orange-peel test is perhaps the most accurate one, although the cold feel and the tendency of the flesh not to go down immediately when pinched are other indications.

The other point about going to a professional is that you will be asked questions about high blood pressure, varicose veins or any other conditions which could be affected by the essential oils. If these do not apply to you, then of course there is no need to worry. But as a general precaution, any cellulite sufferer who also has other health problems, such as fluid retention, arthritis, high blood pressure, a heart condition, or any other serious illness, would be advised to seek professional help.

Usually, though, cellulite is a condition which is unaccompanied by any other illness. Most cellulite victims feel perfectly well and healthy, and have no idea that their bodies may be loaded down with toxic material.

Do Patent Anti-Cellulite Treatments Work?

In a word, no. There is no cream or oil on the market which will magically melt away cellulite, nor is there likely to be. Most chemists' shops and department-store beauty counters are full of creams and lotions which purport to firm up flabby areas and improve body contours. Don't fall for them, especially as some of the ones on the market these days cost £20 or more for a small jar. Whatever cream, oil or lotion you buy, you will be wasting your money completely unless you are also prepared to go on the diet and undertake daily body brushing.

Professor Sam Shuster, who is convinced that cellulite is a load of cobblers, does not believe that there is any cream on the market which can get rid of fat. He said in an interview with Maggie Drummond in *The Sunday Times*, June 1988, that any skin cream which got far enough down to have an effect on the body would have to be classed as a drug rather than a cosmetic, and would not be on general sale. These creams can do no more than a brisk walk, a body brush, or a quick rub-down with a loofah after a bath would do.

Just recently one or two aromatherapy-based anti-cellulite oils have come onto the market. One is available at branches of The Body Shop, another is manufactured by Bodytreats, a specialist aromatherapy company. The Neals Yard apothecary shop in London also sells a special anti-cellulite oil.

These oils should always be used in conjunction with the programme outlined above, not just by themselves. But they are not, like the creams from major cosmetic houses, an expensive waste of money. They can work, but only together with the other treatments, and only if you apply them regularly and properly – there's nothing, unfortunately, which will make cellulite go away without hard work from you. This applies even if you decide to put your thighs into the care of a professional therapist.

In the end, there's only one person who can make the cellulite disappear, and that's you.

How Do I Embark on an Anti-Cellulite Programme?

The best way is gradually. Although the programme is extremely beneficial to health generally, it has to be realized that a toxic body takes time to heal itself. The more toxic the system is, the longer any cleansing programme will take.

Also, the body may react unfavourably at first to a drastic change in diet, however healthy this may be. We are primarily creatures of habit, and our bodies get used to whatever foods and drinks we give them. They may rebel when anything is withdrawn suddenly.

If you smoke, drink a lot of alcohol, eat junk foods, down several cups of coffee a day, and are also extremely sedentary it is unrealistic to suppose that you can revert to good habits in a single day. You will not be able to give up all your props and addictions at once, as this will represent too drastic a change for your system to handle. Also, you may well feel extremely deprived, and as if life is not worth living. It is only when people become released from their addictions and cravings that they come to realize that life is actually *more* enjoyable without the artificial props.

Those who smoke should make giving up or cutting down an urgent priority, long before they embark on the anti-cellulite regime. The difficulty of giving up smoking should never be underestimated. On the other hand, there is little point in undertaking the diet and the body brushing if you continue to smoke twenty or more cigarettes a day.

Once you have successfully conquered smoking, the next priority is to try to give up coffee and tea. Again, these beverages can form potent addictions, and be extremely hard to renounce. As one who has tried to give up both cigarettes and caffeine – though not at the same time – I can say that caffeine is definitely easier than nicotine. Nicotine is one of the most addictive drugs available – and one of the hardest to get out of the system.

Once you have managed to give up smoking, tea and coffee, then it will be time to embark on the anti-cellulite diet. This has to be very strict for two weeks, after which time it can be modified. You can even have the occasional cup of tea and coffee.

Once you start the diet you can consider that you have started the anti-cellulite regime proper. At the same time as beginning the diet, do the body brushing, the massage and the rubbing-in of essential oils.

You will find that after a very short time you will feel quite different about yourself. The first effect you will notice is that you go to the lavatory far more. You may also find that your skin breaks out in acne, that you get more earwax, and that your skin becomes very dry. You will probably also discover that you sweat more. These are all signs that the regime is working.

Those with extremely toxic systems may find themselves feeling rather unwell for three or four days. They may experience headaches, nausea, a sensation of disorientation, mood swings. All these will pass in about a week, at most.

How Long Before the Cellulite Starts to Go?

This depends on how strict you are with yourself and how much cellulite you have in the first place.

Most therapists reckon that six of their treatments – if possible two a week – combined with diet and brushing at home, will rid thighs of cellulite. In my own case it took far longer, but then I had suffered a severe cellulite problem for two decades. Patricia Davis says that she has never met anybody who needs more than ten treatments. You will certainly find that the cellulite starts to go after two weeks of the regime.

Before starting, measure your thighs at the thickest part, and note down the measurement. Then, as you proceed with the programme, measure your thighs weekly, to see if there is any difference. There will certainly be a measurable loss after about a month.

If, after two weeks, you don't seem to be getting anywhere, don't give up hope. There is no cellulite in the world that can withstand the regime detailed in this book – so long as you follow it conscientiously and regularly. It is the *regularity of the treatments which does the trick. Nothing will work if it is remembered only occasionally.*

Anti-Cellulite Programme

PRE-PROGRAMME

Cut Out — *Cut Down*
Smoking — Alcohol
Coffee

PROGRAMME

Take Up
Detoxifying diet for
  two weeks
Dry skin brushing daily
  before bath
Massage using aromatherapy
  oils *after* bath

POST-PROGRAMME

Keep Up
Exercise for toning
Healthy diet
Skin brushing twice a week
Occasional massage

CHAPTER FOUR

THE ANTI-CELLULITE DIET

All restricted food-intake diets are tough, and the anti-cellulite diet is no exception. But for anybody who really wants to get rid of the lumps and bumps it's not an optional extra but an absolute necessity.

So many of us imagine that it would be really lovely to be able to eat and drink exactly what we like and not get fat, unhealthy, suffer from hangovers or develop cellulite. Unfortunately, the foods that we come to love and crave are usually those that the body least wants, and finds hardest to digest.

So there's nothing for it but to make up your mind to become spartan and abstemious, at least until the cellulite has gone – and even afterwards, if you want it to stay away. Because like household dust, mice, greenfly on roses and ants, cellulite is always threatening to come back, and will do so at the very least opportunity.

I found that the best way to brainwash myself into sticking to the diet was to see myself as an ill person for whom the diet was a sure way to start getting better. It always helps if you can have a positive attitude, as that is what keeps you going, in the end.

The diet advocated here is the one first developed by Dr Weston Price, a dentist who went round the world recording the diet of people in pre-literate societies. He discovered time and again that the closer to nature their food, the healthier they stayed. The 'primitive' diets eaten by these people appeared to be the real key to their continuing good health. From this Dr Price concluded that the more removed from nature a diet was, the worse the general health of any community became. The more people ate white bread, chips, salted peanuts, crisps, and processed foods, the more they suffered from ill-health.

Over the years, Dr Price's ideas were taken up by other doctors and nutritionists who, until the 1980s, remained mainly on the fringes and were considered extremely cranky and peculiar. It wasn't until people such as health writer Leslie Kenton, nutritionists Celia Wright and Patrick Holford, and Dr Alan Stewart of the British Society for Nutritional Medicine, began writing about these diets in popular magazines that they gained general acceptance.

I say 'acceptance' but of course, the 'healthy' diet still is not accepted by everybody as the main ingredient of lasting health. Some authorities still laugh at the idea of 'detoxifying' and clearing the system of poisons by a pure diet. But the monastic, detoxifying diet is what health farms all over the world have been advocating for the past hundred years at least. Health farms were originally set up for the purpose of detoxifying over-indulgent Victorians whose lavish, eight-course meals laden with fats and meats had led to obesity and a number of degenerative diseases.

It is only since the mid-1970s that the natural detoxifying

diet has been put forward as the best way to start getting rid of cellulite. Now it has been eagerly adopted by all therapists who treat these lumps and bumps, and their grateful clients know that they owe their newly cellulite-free limbs in large part to following the recommended diet.

The first step in any cellulite-removing regime is a thorough cleansing of the system. The more clogged up the body is, the more drastic the cleansing will have to be. If it is really bad you may do well to eat nothing but fruit and vegetables, raw whenever possible, for about two weeks. This gives the liver and lymphatic system a chance to unclog and to start working efficiently once more to expel the accumulated wastes. When eating a fruit-only diet, you should stick to one variety at each meal. That is, only bananas, only grapes, or only apples, for example. The reason for this is that different fruits have different acid levels and may interfere with each other.

As mentioned in the previous chapter, you really have to cut out tea and coffee, ideally drinking neither for at least two weeks. Now, very many people find that cutting out tea and coffee is quite the hardest part of the diet. This is because over the years they have become addicted to them, usually quite without realizing it.

Coffee, as we have seen, is a potent cellulite-causer, and the same goes for all caffeine-loaded drinks – tea, chocolate, colas – even the calorie-free variety. Don't drink these either while you are trying to rid yourself of cellulite.

When attempting to cut out tea and coffee you will soon know if you are addicted. Try going without either of them for forty-eight hours, and see how you feel when drinking herbal substitutes instead. If you are used to drinking more than three cups of tea or coffee in a single day you will most probably experience quite severe withdrawal symptoms. These, say many doctors, can be quite as bad as withdrawing from heroin.

Caffeine is a potent drug, and its sudden withdrawal temporarily upsets the system, causing very bad migraine headaches and a feeling of disorientation. In my case the migraine I suffered from sudden caffeine withdrawal was so bad that I had to go to bed. I simply couldn't work. In addition, I felt miserable and depressed. Assured that these symptoms would pass in time, I waited and waited. It took about a week for the worst of the symptoms to wear off, but I never really felt well while not drinking any tea or coffee.

In the end, my therapist sympathized and advised me to go back to one cup of real coffee a day, so long as it was made with freshly ground beans that were kept in the freezer to ensure freshness. I did, and instantly my spirits lifted. Now I drink just that one delicious, not-to-be-missed cup of coffee a day, and have one cup of Luaka or ordinary tea in the afternoon. But on an anti-cellulite regime the coffee you drink must be real, made from freshly ground beans. You should not under any circumstances drink the instant variety, as this not only has caffeine added but is made by a high-tech process which renders it completely artificial.

At the same time as cutting down on tea or coffee, it is important to increase considerably your intake of mineral water. Any mineral water on the market will do, but try not to drink tap water too much. When starting the cleansing regime, you should drink as many as eight glasses of mineral water a day, if you can remember to do so. In my case, I found constant Perrier and Badoit so boring that I kept forgetting to drink them. For me, the carbonated drinks are slightly more interesting and fun to drink than the still ones, although not much. Some people have said that they can get 'high' on Perrier, and there is at least one recent study to show that if people believe they are drinking alcohol when they are not, they can still get tipsy.

While on the subject of getting tipsy, it is important to avoid all alcohol, if possible, when on the initial cleansing programme. Alcohol has a similar effect on body metabolism to caffeine, in that it raises blood sugar content instantly, and then the body has to work hard to accommodate the extra glucose. As with caffeine, it tends to end up in fat stores eventually. Also, taking alcohol whilst on a cleansing diet tends to overload the liver, which is now having to work overtime anyway to eliminate all the waste matter rapidly being freed from cellulite-loaded areas.

Fruit juices can be drunk in moderation, and preferably diluted with mineral water, as 'neat' they can be too strong for a system in the process of detoxification. Look out for the natural brands, such as Copella or Aspall, which are made with real fruits instead of concentrates. Of course, avoid all sugar-laden fruit drinks and squashes.

Now we come on to the thorny subject of food. Ideally, all your food should be raw, organically grown, eaten the day of purchase, or picked from your own garden, unfrozen, un-processed, unsalted, unsugared, untreated in any way. Clearly, this kind of diet is virtually impossible for anybody to follow at home, although some health farms specialize in this kind of therapy.

While on the cleansing regime it is also more or less impossible to eat in a restaurant, go out to dinner, or have a quick snack in a café. You have to make up your mind to be an unsociable hermit, so it is best to pick a fortnight when you have few social or work engagements. It may seem hard, and the ultimate in deprivation, but if you keep reminding yourself that the whole purpose of the cleansing regime is to give the cellulite deposits a reasonable chance of dispersing, you will be encouraged to continue.

Some people with really bad cellulite are put on a fruit juice fast for a few days, to ensure that the worst of the toxins are eliminated quickly. I found I could not exist on the fast, because I was too busy and active all the time. Most diet books which advocate fasting advise you to pick days when you are not doing much more than mooching around at home. But very few of us in reality have days like that. It is a good idea, though, at least to try to eat nothing but fruit and vegetables for that important two weeks. The main idea behind the fruit-and-vegetable-only diet is that these are the foods the body finds easiest to digest. They will not put any kind of strain on the liver or kidneys. The more difficult foods are to digest, the less chance you will have of the cellulite disappearing. You can't expect the organs of elimination to be able to do everything at once. Anything processed, cooked or generally denatured adds to the burden on the digestive system.

Some people allege that they feel wonderful straightaway on an all-fruit-and-vegetable diet. Many more will feel quite

terrible at first. This is mainly because the body takes time to
adapt to any radical change of diet. This applies even if you
are changing from an unhealthy to an extremely healthy
diet. So you should be prepared for some feelings of disorientation and discomfort, for cravings, depression and bad
temper, at first. These are all withdrawal symptoms, a sign
that something is happening, and they won't last for more
than a few days.

Another reason why an all-plant-food diet can cause initial
problems is that we tend to underestimate the sheer force of
habit. Many people embarking on a stringent diet for the first
time simply are not prepared for the drastic body changes that
might happen. You will certainly find changes in bowel
movements and frequency of urination. You may also find
that you sweat more, and may erupt in the kind of spots you
haven't had since adolescence. Some women also experience menstrual changes.

In my case I found that initially, apart from headaches, I
suffered from insomnia, which is unusual for me. Not only
that, but my nights were disturbed by visions of wonderful
toast dripping with butter, cups of coffee, meals in rest-
aurants and so on. In his searing book on concentration
camps, *If This is a Man*, Primo Levi writes about how the
inmates used to dream about food night after night. Something similar may happen when you first embark on an
all-fruit-and-vegetable diet. If it does, it's just withdrawal
symptoms, not a sign that you are chronically malnourished,
as the concentration camp victims were. You may also feel
rather miserable for no apparent reason, and this is again a
sign that you are suffering from withdrawal. Don't forget that

butter, cream, bread and cakes can be quite as addictive as any drugs – and sudden deprivation may have a marked effect.

None of these symptoms is anything to worry about; they are simply indications that the body is at last getting rid of toxic wastes. To add insult to injury, it is extremely unlikely that you will notice any difference in the cellulite at first. It will usually be a week or two before the stuff even begins to shift.

Although the initial cleansing diet consists of fruit and vegetables, don't imagine that any old fruit and veg will do. Far from it. Even here, you have to be careful. Citrus fruits such as oranges and grapefruit are out except very occasionally, as they are rather rough on the liver. But definitely in are bananas, apples, pears, pineapple, all the exotica such as mangoes, papaya, passion fruit, sharon fruit (the hard, orange-coloured fruits which come from Israel), kiwi fruit, grapes, strawberries (very good – especially English ones), raspberries, blackberries. If you are eating fruit alone for the first few days you can eat almost any amount – up to six pounds a day. You should eat some fruit every two hours, otherwise you will start to feel hungry, and should drink plenty of mineral water in between. Most nutritional experts do not advise eating and drinking together, as water dilutes the digestive juices.

Good vegetables are: potatoes, spinach, cauliflower, broccoli, cabbage, mangetout, beans, turnips, swedes, green peppers, carrots, celery. Not all of these can be eaten raw, of course, but wherever possible, eat without cooking. Spinach, cauliflower and broccoli are delicious raw, with a small amount of vinaigrette or lemon dressing. Again, the portions of raw vegetables can be as large as you like.

People who are not used to eating like this, or who have never been to a health farm where this kind of diet is standard, will find it very peculiar. Do try to persevere, though, as it will really get the cellulite shifting when combined with body-brushing and the other treatments.

Here is a typical day's eating and drinking plan for the first two weeks on an anti-cellulite regime:

ON RISING
A glass of hot water with a small amount of lemon, or one of the 'wake-up' herb teas such as Early Morn, or a glass of cold water. Always use mineral rather than tap water for early morning drinks if you can.

BREAKFAST
A couple of bananas, apples, or a huge bunch of grapes. That's it. Plus, of course, mineral water either half an hour before or half an hour after the fruit.

Those who know that they are simply not going to be able to manage on fruit alone should not reach for the nearest slice of bread, but should nibble sunflower, sesame or pumpkin seeds. If you have a coffee grinder, grind up equal amounts of these seeds and sprinkle them on the fruit. Then you won't feel hungry, although it may be difficult at first not to eat that really delicious toast, butter and marmalade that the others are tucking into.

MID-MORNING

Eat more fruit if you are at home. If at work, take a selection of fruit and seeds with you. Bananas are particularly good at assuaging hunger.

LUNCH

Whenever possible, eat a large salad consisting of raw vegetables. Carrots, cauliflower and broccoli are all quite filling, and you can eat as much of them as you like. Those who are not used to raw vegetables may find eating them very odd at first, although they are becoming more accepted nowadays. If you can't be bothered to cut and chop your own, Marks and Spencer now do some wonderful ready-prepared salads which come complete with dressings. Although these bought salads may seem expensive, they can actually work out cheaper than buying whole cauliflowers, pounds of carrots, broccoli, etc, which you may have a job to finish before they start going off.

MID-AFTERNOON

Have a cup of herb tea or Luaka if you are feeling like crawling up the wall by now, and some more fruit. Throughout the day, drink lots of mineral water, but not too many herb teas. Some of them can be quite strong.

SUPPER

Here you can have some vegetable soup, sprinkled with ground seeds, and then another huge vegetable salad, or just some more fruit if you can manage it.

BEFORE BED

You'll be sick to death of fruit and vegetables by now, and anyway they don't seem to be very good last thing at night. If you really feel you must have something before retiring, have an oatcake, or an organic rice cake thinly covered with sesame seed spread. As a bedtime drink you can try Barley-cup. Some people like this drink but I could never get used to it. If you haven't had too many cups of herb tea throughout the day, have one now, formulated for late at night. An 'early-morning' herb tea at this time may keep you awake.

Note: When embarking on this diet, you may find it difficult to get to sleep. This is partly because you are changing your eating habits radically and your body has not adjusted to them, and partly because you are feeling deprived of tea and coffee. A bedtime herb drink will help you get over insomnia which in any case should not last for too long. It all depends on how poisoned your system is and for how long you have been eating a denatured diet.

Those who find this diet impossible should cook a large quantity of brown rice and keep it in the fridge to turn to when, and if, hunger becomes acute and painful. Actually, the problems don't lie so much with actual hunger as with the fact that you are not now eating any of the comforting foods.

When starting the anti-cellulite diet you have to give priority to this form of eating. It is not a good idea to do it at the same time as moving house, starting a new job, or undergoing any emotional or physical upheavals. Getting rid of the cellulite is hard work and upheaval enough, and you should, ideally, concentrate on this task alone for a time.

After ten days to two weeks you can introduce a wider variety of foods to your diet. You can start off in the morning with porridge or muesli, in both cases not made with milk. Muesli can be soaked overnight in a little mineral water or fruit juice and eaten with yogurt in the morning – so long as it's natural, low-fat, live yoghurt and not of the thick and creamy variety. You can eat oatcakes spread with sesame or sunflower seed paste, or a margarine such as Vitaquell. Tofu, a cheese-like substance made from soya flour, is a very good substitute for milk, cream and cheese and is a wonderfully adaptable food. And you can now have that most marvellous treat, a cup of real coffee every single day.

While on the regime, avoid all dairy products as much as possible. You can make nut 'cream' which is almost (although not quite) as good as double cream, from simply blending together cashew nuts or almonds, a little honey and enough water to give pouring consistency. Your best friend now is not diamonds, but a food processor. In fact, I would almost say that this gadget is essential for anybody on an anti-cellulite diet.

If you have the occasional lapse during the first two weeks' anti-cellulite diet, at least make sure that you have a big salad at every main meal. To some extent, this will neutralize the bad effect of anything else you might have eaten.

Two of the best kinds of food for anybody wishing to keep cellulite away for ever are nuts and pulses. Those who are vegetarian or who have drastically reduced their meat and fish intake may worry about getting enough protein, although you do not have to worry about this until the initial two weeks are up – you'll have plenty of stored fats to keep you going. Nuts and pulses provide plenty of protein. At one time it was difficult to buy a variety of pulses but now lentils of all colours, soya beans, flageolets, blackeye beans, red and black kidney beans, mung beans and split peas are on sale at practically all supermarkets. You can also easily buy brazils, almonds and cashew nuts – all manna to the cellulite shifter.

Pulses and nuts are very versatile. You can put them into soups, stews, curries and salads, or make them into pâtés, and they will keep you feeling pleasantly full for hours. Pulses can be flavoured with fresh ginger and herbs and eaten with brown rice. As time goes on, you will experience new taste sensations. Many people who have been on a detox-ifying and cleansing diet for any length of time find they simply can't go back to their old ways. Cakes, white pastry, thick cream and biscuits start to taste heavy and cloying. You can almost sense the cellulite going back on if you bite into one of these products.

Don't imagine, though, that you have to say goodbye to these foods for ever. The occasional slice of Black Forest gâteau or dish swimming in cream sauce does you no harm at all, and if you find it absolutely delicious, it probably does you good psychologically, too. I remember in the thick of my own detoxifying diet I felt ravenous during the interval of a concert at the Royal Festival Hall. As usual, there was nothing I could eat and, in desperation, I had just one Cornetto. I can't remember when I've enjoyed anything quite so much. It was absolutely wonderful – but I didn't crave another Cornetto for months and months afterwards. That one little treat was enough.

It is a good idea to keep a food and drink diary at this stage to record exactly what you are eating, and to monitor good and bad reactions to food. You may discover that the days seem very long without tea or coffee, and particularly if you are used to drinking alcohol at every meal. You will almost certainly miss chocolate, cocoa, cream, cheese, bread and butter at first. Think of them not as delicious foods, but as poisons which all add to the cellulite load – then it will be easier to avoid them.

Until the cellulite goes, you should avoid all white flour and refined products. This goes for white rice, white pasta, all shop-bought cakes and biscuits, white bread and rolls. Instead, you can buy buckwheat spaghetti, wholemeal macaroni and other pasta, brown rice and wholemeal bread. Dried fruit can be eaten in moderation, and is best soaked overnight. You will probably find you become an *aficionado* of the local health food shop and, before very long, an expert on healthy foods.

Very attractive breakfasts and desserts can be made by blending together in a food processor soaked dried fruit such as hunza apricots, a small amount of natural yoghurt, a squeeze of lemon and real honey. Some honeys, particularly the ones that are the 'produce of several countries', are not the real thing at all, but highly processed. As one might expect, it is the more expensive honeys that are likely to be the best ones. As so little is eaten at one time, it is worth buying the better brands.

As a committed vegetarian myself, I naturally do not

advocate eating fish and meat. I must say that vegetarianism *per se* made not the slightest difference to my cellulite. I did get thinner, but the cellulite stayed firmly in place, blast it. But for non-vegetarian cellulite removers, occasional fish or meat does no harm. Most fish, I understand, is not artificially fed and reared, but ideally you should avoid all meats which have been intensively farmed, such as turkey, chicken and pork. Lamb is usually all right, and is, in fact, one of the better meats you can get today. Beef is often full of antibiotics and should be eaten only occasionally. You can now buy additive-free meat – butchers who sell this advertise it as such.

Celia Wright, author of the excellent book *The Wright Diet*, which forms the basis for the anti-cellulite diet advocated by most therapists, strongly advises against eating pork in any form. She says that almost all pork is infected with a parasite called *trichinosis*, which is easily passed to humans. Also bacon, sausages, tinned, frozen and preserved meats should not be eaten by anybody serious about keeping cellulite off. All these products are likely to contain high amounts of salt, other preservatives, and artificial colours and are usually highly processed into the bargain. Those who have a cellulite problem should, ideally, avoid processed and artificial foods altogether for the rest of their lives. However, you should not try to give everything up at once. This is patently impossible.

The good news about alcohol is that, after the first booze-free fortnight of the serious anti-cellulite regime, you can gradually introduce the occasional drink back into your life. In fact, if you can drink only organic wines, they will even do you good. Wines with additives, such as sugar and chemicals, may not do the system any good, but the organic ones actually help digestion.

To sum up, you should avoid, at least for the first fortnight of anti-cellulite eating: bread and butter, milk and dairy products, meat and fish if possible, all processed foods, anything cooked, salted nuts and crisps, all preserved meats, spirits, smoked foods, instant coffee (best to avoid this at all times, anyway), and ready-frozen meals. All these substances are cellulite-forming and will undo all the good work you are doing in other areas.

Also best avoided are all products made with white or refined flour, bread, biscuits, ice-cream, pastry, bought sauces, pasta, and all fried foods.

One of the earliest signs that the cellulite is starting to go is that you urinate much more frequently. Indeed, as the system starts to shake itself up, you may find you are going to the toilet up to three times before breakfast. Also, on the fruit diet you will find a definite increase in bowel movements. This, too, indicates that cellulite is starting to shift.

Books such as Leslie and Susannah Kenton's *Raw Energy* and Celia Wright's *The Wright Diet* give more detailed information on eating the all-fruit-and-vegetable diet. If you can manage it for a whole two weeks then you will be well on the way towards shifting that awful cellulite. And, as a plus, your general health will improve by leaps and bounds as well.

CHAPTER FIVE

DRY SKIN BRUSHING

I first came across the concept of dry skin brushing in Dr Robert Gray's *The Colon Health Handbook*, where he recommended five minutes' skin brushing a day in order to cleanse the lymphatic system and get it working efficiently once more.

Body brushing, he explained, is a very effective way of enabling the lymphatic system to clear itself and expel waste material which has been held for a long time inside the body. In addition this technique can correct inflammations of the lymph nodes. In order to be really effective, any skin-brushing programme must be kept up for several months, and it is important to use a special kind of brush which has particularly hard and scratchy bristles.

When I first read that scouring yourself all over with a dry, scratchy brush could tone up the whole internal system I found it hard to believe. How could brushing yourself on the outside make any difference to what happened inside your body? Back brushes and loofahs have long been a standard part of bathroom equipment, but the idea that the brushing could activate internal organs sounded very suspect indeed, just one more of those crazy Californian notions which were being put about in the early 1980s.

Of course, Robert Gray was only talking about the power of skin brushing to help the colon to clear. His book did not mention cellulite at all, and it was to be several years before skin brushing was advocated for cellulite removal. But not long after reading Robert Gray's book, I began to hear more and more about the benefits of dry skin brushing. A number of alternative practitioners in Britain soon became extremely enthusiastic about it and were advising their patients to brush themselves daily before having their bath, as it was all wonderfully stimulating and would help you feel alive and awake, as well as releasing new levels of energy.

As time went on, enormous benefits were being claimed for dry skin brushing. I don't know who invented, or developed, the technique, but it rapidly became extremely respectable among practitioners of complementary therapies. Orthodox doctors, of course, laughed it to scorn.

As soon as aromatherapists and other practitioners who were trying to treat cellulite heard about the technique they felt certain it could be of enormous use in getting rid of the toxins which cause the lumpy deposits. They tried it out, and soon discovered that it was just as effective in dispersing cellulite as it was supposed to be in helping to cleanse the colon. As both conditions were caused, above all, by a sluggish lymphatic system, anything which could help one problem would almost certainly be efficacious for the other. Body brushing soon caught on because it was, above all, cheap and easy to do. It did not require expensive equipment, and anybody could learn how to do it very quickly.

Nowadays, enthusiasts are claiming that the technique has many benefits apart from its ability to remove cellulite or clean out colons. Skin brushing can tone up your whole system, encourage ordinary fat cells to disperse, invigorate the brain and also remove stress and tension from the system, according to its advocates. In a very few short years, body brushing has become a standard technique recommended by those doctors, nutritionists and healers who are interested in natural healing rather than relying on drugs, surgery and hospitals.

Another American expert, Dr Jack Soltanoff, author of *Natural Healing*, reckons that just five minutes' skin brushing a day can improve digestion, aid metabolism and impart new levels of energy – as well as get rid of cellulite. In his book he writes:

The technique is a mild form of acupressure and acupuncture performed without piercing the skin. The only tool that is required is a scrub or handbrush. When followed correctly and in the proper sequence, the dry friction skin bath has far-reaching beneficial effects on your health because it affects all the inner organs in the remote parts of your body via the reflexes of the nervous system.

As your skin and circulation are affected, the technique produces a wonderful feeling and a warm glow . . . The dry skin friction bath is extremely beneficial for those whose office jobs force them to sit at a desk all day, and especially those who must sit in rigid or cramped positions in front of computer terminals or typewriters day after day.

Dr Soltanoff considers that the other eliminative organs, such as the bowels, lungs and kidneys, are abused daily by most of us with the overconsumption of 'refined, commercialized processed foods, tobaccos, coffee, tea, chocolate, alcohol'. The skin-brushing technique has the power, he says, to stimulate these organs into eliminating effectively.

On the ability of skin brushing to disperse cellulite, Dr Soltanoff writes:

This technique works on cellulite by gradually breaking down the obese liquid-filled fatty tissues and slowly releasing the toxic fluids through various channels, particularly the lymphatic system. With regular daily use, your legs will firm up and tighten. You'll have a much younger figure, and that in itself will make you feel terrific.

Skin brushing seems like a fairly passive activity, in that it can be carried out in your own bathroom, but some advocates believe that it can even replace jogging. A number of American natural-health experts are now saying that five minutes of the right kind of body brushing a day is as good as half an hour's pounding the streets. You don't get the aerobic effect of course, but the benefits to your circulation and digestive system are as great.

The technique can also retard the ageing process of the skin, greatly improve your figure, and even enable you to banish apathy and boredom, say some American practitioners. Dr Soltanoff is such an enthusiast for daily body brushing that he maintains it is possible literally to brush all your troubles away – mental, physical and even emotional ones.

Dr Soltanoff, a chiropractor who recommends the skin-brushing technique to all of his patients, believes along with Dr Robert Gray that there is no better way of activating and cleansing the lymphatic system. The skin, he says, is the largest eliminative organ in the body and when it doesn't function properly, an enormous burden is placed on all other eliminative organs, such as the bowels, lungs and kidneys. They have to work far harder than they should. In an average day, says Dr Soltanoff, the skin will eliminate as much waste matter as the kidneys or lungs. The trouble is that for most of us the skin has become clogged up too, and is less efficient as an organ of elimination than it ought to be because the pores cannot get rid of waste products properly. This means they stay in the system and add to the burden of waste material which eventually leads to cellulite and other problems caused by faulty elimination of rubbish.

Kitty Campion, a British herbalist who became converted to body brushing in the early 1980s, now uses it on many patients who go to her clinic near Stoke-on-Trent. 'When you first try it out,' she warns, 'skin brushing feels very strange and unusual. It's rather scratchy and uncomfortable, if you use the correct kind of brush, and is not at all the same sensation as brushing with a loofah, for instance. But though it seems so new, in fact the technique of skin brushing for health has been known for thousands of years. We are rediscovering it, rather than inventing something new. I find that most people wonder however they managed without it, once they get used to it.'

Kitty Campion says that many people who come to her for herbal treatments are in very poor health, even if they are not always aware of this. 'A common condition these days is that the kidneys and lungs are not functioning as well as they should. They have become sluggish, and inefficient at eliminating waste material. I usually recommend skin brushing to all my clients, as a first step on their way back to health. It sounds odd to say that just by brushing, you can activate internal systems and get them working again, but that's exactly what happens.'

She lists the benefits of skin brushing in her book, A Woman's Herbal. Firstly, daily brushing removes the dead layers of skin and other impurities, allowing the pores to eliminate without obstruction. Secondly, the technique stimulates circulation, so that the blood nourishing those organs of the body which lie near the surface reaches them effectively. Thirdly, it is an excellent way of removing cellulite and clearing the lymphatic system.

The main benefit, though, according to Kitty Campion, is that it helps to prevent premature ageing and induces a wonderful sense of well-being. She writes: 'Many of my patients complain a lot about the things I ask them to do but I have never yet encountered one who has complained about skin scrubbing. Once they get used to it, they love it!'

If you want to see for yourself just how many dead cells fly off when skin brushing, says Kitty, brush in bright sunlight and you'll see huge amounts of dust coming off.

Frances Clifford, the aromatherapist who successfully

helped me to get rid of two decades of cellulite deposits, is also extremely enthusiastic about dry skin brushing. She says, 'Body brushing is wonderful for sloughing off dead skin cells. It stimulates blood flow and gets oxygen to all parts of the body. The technique strengthens the immune system as well, and is extremely good for anybody suffering from low energy levels. I do skin brushing now on all my clients, and they love it, because it makes them feel so good.'

It was after investigating the benefits of dry skin brushing for myself that I bought a brush and gave the technique a try. I must say that I hated it at first. The brush was so very scratchy, and I could only apply very light pressure. Also, it hurt a lot when I stepped into the bath right after brushing my skin. But I persevered and soon got used to it. My skin started to welcome the daily brushing. After a few weeks, I started to enjoy it and then missed it if I didn't do it for any reason.

I now have no doubt whatever that skin brushing played a major part in enabling my own cellulite to disappear, and so I can heartily recommend the practice from personal experience. It can do you no possible harm, and will only do good, so long as you never break the skin when brushing.

It is essential to have the correct type of brush. This must be very hard, and made of natural, not synthetic fibres. A soft bristle brush won't have the same effect at all. Most body brushing experts recommend a long-handled brush made of Mexican cactus fibre. The handle should be detachable, and made of natural wood, with a strap across the brush.

These brushes are very stiff and scratchy when you first use them, and you may feel that they will take your skin off. If yours scratches too much, soak it for a few hours in the bathroom basin, then dry overnight in the airing cupboard. It will then be soft enough to use without harming the skin.

In order for dry skin brushing to be really effective, the strokes you apply have to be firm and long. Start with light pressure and gradually build up, as your skin becomes used to the sensation. You will discover in time that the skin can take quite hard pressure, but it will probably be tender at first.

Dry skin brushing in this way is not the same thing as rubbing your skin with a loofah, bath mitt or ordinary back brush. None of these will work to break down cellulite, or activate the lymphatic system because they go soft very quickly. It is only all-over brushing with the right kind of brush which will have this effect.

If you are interested only in brushing to get rid of cellulite, you can just concentrate on these areas. The pressure can be as hard as you like. Brush up the back of the leg in long, single strokes (see diagram). Then when you get to the thigh, brush upwards as vigorously as you can where the cellulite is at its most dense. Finish off by brushing the buttocks equally hard,

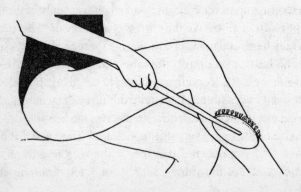

in any direction. Usually, skin brushing has to be done in the direction of the heart, but circular movements round the buttocks are best.

Brush both legs an equal amount and then get into the bath. You will find that the bath water makes your skin tingle pleasantly. If you are doing body brushing in conjunction with aromatherapy you should rub in the essential oils straight after you get out of the bath, again paying particular attention to the cellulite areas. The best time for applying the massage oils is after body brushing and a bath because then the pores will be open and unclogged. Kitty Campion advises a short, cold shower after a long, hot bath to maximize the effect of skin scrubbing, but not everybody will be able to stand the invigorating effect of this treatment. From a cellulite-removing point of view, there is no need to add the cold shower to the range of treatments.

If you find the brushing has left long scratches, or makes you look as though you had walked through a field of brambles, you are either doing it too hard or the brush needs more soaking. The brushing should never be allowed to break the skin. In any case, never brush over broken skin.

The Whole-Body Brush

You don't, of course, have to limit skin brushing to cellulite-dense areas. A whole-body brush will tone up the system even more, and increase the benefits.

This is how to do it.

You should start by brushing your fingers and hands. Hold

your hand with fingers splayed, and brush between each finger a few times. Brush on top of the hand and then the palm, as many times as you like. Repeat this with the other hand.

Now do your arms. Brush in long strokes from the wrist to the elbow, then from the elbow to the shoulder. Always use long, firm, bold strokes, and remember always to brush in the direction of the heart.

After this, do your toes and feet. Put one leg on the rim of the bath or basin, and brush across the tops of the toes. Brush the soles of the feet, then around the ankles. Again, use the firmest possible strokes. Brush the leg up to the knee, going all round the leg and using long strokes from the ankle. Repeat this about fourteen times. Now brush the thighs and buttocks. Repeat with the other leg. As you brush, you will soon get to know the cellulite areas, and you will see them gradually diminishing over the weeks. But don't expect that one vigorous brushing session will send them away. For really bad cellulite, you may have to keep this practice up for several months. Anybody who wishes to stop the cellulite coming back – as it will always try to do – should build body brushing into their everyday lives.

After having a real good go at the worst areas of cellulite you should now move up to the neck. Brush downwards from the head, front and back. Now do the shoulders, this time brushing downwards, to keep in the direction of the heart.

Cellulite sufferers can help to activate the lymphatic system by holding the brush in the armpit and rotating it seven times to the left and seven times to the right. This action, if repeated daily, gets the lymph nodes working again.

Women who visit an aromatherapist for the removal of cellulite will discover that the therapist always does this towards the end of a treatment.

Now do the front and sides of the body. Women should avoid brushing over the nipples, but can brush over the breasts, perhaps with lighter pressure. Some authorities do not advise brushing over the stomach and abdomen, as the action can be too strong. It is probably better to leave this area alone, and go on to the back. You will need the long handle to reach the back and again, long, firm strokes should be employed.

Although this procedure may sound complicated, in fact it is very simple indeed and takes no more than five minutes per session. Women with very bad cellulite should spend at least five minutes a day on body brushing for two months. After this length of time, the body gets used to the brushing and the technique is less effective. When this has happened, you should brush every other day. Kitty Campion says, 'The idea is to surprise your skin. Skin brushing is subject, as is the use of herbs, to homeostatic resistance – that is, your skin will get used to it and stop responding so well.' She suggests juggling the days of the week around, so that your skin does not always know when it is going to get the treatment. Other therapists I have spoken to confirm the fact that skin brushing loses its efficacy after a time, and that breaks have to be built into the treatment.

Some women find that once they start on a serious anti-cellulite regime they can't stop, and tend to overdo it at first. But the body has to be helped to get rid of its cellulite gently and safely, and you have to be patient. Just because five minutes of body brushing is good, it doesn't follow that ten minutes or quarter of an hour will be much better. Be gentle at first, and build up pressure gradually once your skin has got used to the sensation.

You may find that your skin does funny things when you embark on brushing it. Remember that this is not just a beauty treatment but an actual health-promoting regime. Most people find that their skin changes texture after a few weeks of brushing. In my case it went extremely dry for a time, and all the massage oils in the world didn't seem to make any difference. But after this, it seemed to go very smooth and unlined. Those who find that their skin seems to alter should just continue with the brushing. It can't do you any harm.

The technique is safe for everybody, except for those who have damaged, infected or broken skin. People who have eczema, psoriasis or any other skin complaint should not use the brush on affected areas. You can brush where the skin is free from damage, though the technique should also not be used on any areas where you have bad varicose veins.

Dry skin brushing is, of course, equally effective for men and women. Men who know they have sluggish kidneys or livers will definitely benefit from an all-over skin brush every morning. If done first thing in the morning it will give a wonderful wake-up sensation.

Some people have even found that dry skin brushing can actually help them to reverse quite serious illnesses. Val Harrod, a British Telecom officer from Stoke-on-Trent, had suffered from an undiagnosed and quite serious liver complaint for many years. She went to doctor after doctor but, although her hands and the soles of her feet were extremely yellow, nobody could discover what was wrong. In the end, worried because she often had to take time off work through illness, Val went to see herbalist Kitty Campion. She said: 'I went to Kitty because I could no longer believe what the doctors were telling me. Kitty diagnosed my condition through iridology (where general health is assessed by the condition of the eyes) and said my liver and lymphatic system were almost completely clogged up. Instead of getting rid of waste, I was just retaining it.

'She recommended skin brushing, and showed me how to do it. Of course, I was extremely sceptical at first, but I tried it, and gradually my liver started to clear. The yellowness on my hands and feet disappeared, and my eyes became brighter. My skin became more alive and the waste started to disperse. Now that I realize how effective skin brushing can be I shall certainly do it for the rest of my life. I do have a faulty liver, which will never work properly and will always be liable to clog up. But I know now that regular skin brushing can prevent the problem from building up.'

Val carries out skin brushing every other day for about ten minutes, and says: 'If you've never done skin brushing before, you can get quite a fright as you see the scales coming off your skin in huge amounts. It makes you realize just how clogged up your pores can get. For me, skin brushing doesn't just have a vague beauty benefit. It has actually cured a serious condition, and probably saved my life. In fact, I was told by a nutritionist recently that but for the brushing I would have eventually died in my own poison.'

Of course, regular skin brushing will not cure every serious liver complaint, and it should not be used as a substitute for medical care. But this story confirms what the skin-brushing enthusiasts claim – that the technique is far more than simply a beauty treatment, or something which makes you vaguely 'feel good'. Daily skin brushing can help to stimulate far-reaching changes for the better within the body.

For cellulite removal though, it must be carried out in conjunction with the cleansing diet detailed in the previous chapter. There is no point in working hard to unclog the system from the outside if you are filling it up with rubbish on the inside.

Once the worst of the cellulite has gone, keep it away by occasional skin brushing once or twice a week. You don't want it to start creeping back after all your hard work.

CHAPTER SIX

AROMATHERAPY

Most people regard aromatherapy as nothing more than a pleasantly relaxing beauty treatment. In fact, essential oils, as they are known, have extremely potent healing powers if used in the right way, and can encourage toxic wastes to disperse and be excreted. Far from being a mildly enjoyable indulgence, aromatherapy oils can enable an ill body or a sluggish system to return to a balanced and harmonious state.

Aromatherapy is the only branch of alternative medicine which really understands cellulite and treats it properly. Once we appreciate that the presence of cellulite is a visible indication of imbalance rather than actual fat, then we can begin to appreciate why and how aromatherapy works.

In her book *Aromatherapy: An A–Z* Patricia Davis says that 'aromatherapy is one of the most spectacularly successful forms of treatment for cellulite'.

The reason, I think, why so many people have been extremely cynical about the power of essential oils to reduce cellulite is because this condition is often attributed to overweight. Over the years there have been many claims that this or that cream, lotion or bodywrap could magically melt away fat. And in every single case where any such product has been subjected to independent investigation, its claims have not stood up at all.

Also aromatherapy has in recent years been very much confined to beauty treatments and beauty salons rather than hospitals or doctors' surgeries, which is why we have tended not to take it seriously. In fact, the science of treating illnesses with essential oils goes back thousands of years. The Ancient Greeks and Egyptians knew that many oils distilled from plants possessed potent therapeutic qualities, but the modern science of aromatherapy can be traced to the First World War, when Dr Jean Valnet, a French army surgeon, used essential oils to treat battle injuries and severe burns. He began to realize that the oils could be used to treat many kinds of illnesses, and after the war he used them on psychiatric patients. His book, *The Practice of Aromatherapy*, has become the standard textbook on the subject, and gives very specific details of how certain oils can help to reverse a wide variety of health problems. In everyday medicine, we use essential oils most often in the form of wintergreen ointment for aches and pains and oil of cloves for toothache.

It should be remembered that, until the advent of laboratory-produced chemical medicine this century, just about all remedies were based on plant materials, many of which have extremely powerful properties. Digitalis, derived from foxglove; heroin and morphine, from the opium poppy; and aspirin, from the willow tree, are all examples of strong medicines which come from plants. In modern times, evening primrose oil, aloe vera and ginseng have been advocated for a variety of health problems. And of course, very many plants can kill. Belladonna, from the deadly nightshade, hemlock and aconite are all examples of plants which can be fatal if you ingest them.

So we should not assume that an innocent-looking, exotic-smelling oil in a plain brown bottle has no healing power. In fact, now that people are becoming increasingly disillusioned with many laboratory-produced drugs because of their adverse side effects, there is an enormous upsurge of interest in natural remedies. This is probably the main reason why aromatherapy is now the fastest-growing of all branches of alternative medicine.

The word 'aromatherapy', like the word cellulite, is basically French, which may be why we in English-speaking countries have been slow to recognize it as a genuine branch of medicine. Aromatherapy can be used either as a beauty treatment, or to treat chronic and serious illness. Nowadays, a number of medical doctors in France are using scientific aromatherapy to treat sinus trouble, tonsillitis and catarrh, as well as for wound healing. Recent research at the Pasteur Institute has shown that certain oils can destroy mucus in the throat and elsewhere, and that aromatic oils can also considerably speed up wound healing. In France, a growing number of doctors are now using essential oils in place of laboratory-produced antibiotics, prescribing them as internal medicine, but you have to be medically qualified to prescribe them to be taken internally. Aromatherapists, as distinct from doctors, only ever use the oils for external purposes.

Pierre Franchomme, a French doctor specializing in the use of essential oils to treat serious illnesses, said at a conference in London in 1987, 'All aromatic oils contain positive or negative charges. It is these electrical charges which help to bring about the healing process.' In France, there is now very well-documented evidence that several oils have powerful detoxifying qualities. It is now becoming increasingly accepted that illnesses result when poisons enter the system, in one form or another. When the body does not contain any poisonous material of any kind, whether this is manufactured inside the body, or comes in from outside, it will remain in perfect health.

It is true that aromatherapy treatments will not bring about any kind of weight loss, nor in themselves will they enable actual fat to shift. What they can do, however, is to encourage the accumulated toxic waste contained in fatty cells to disperse and be eliminated through the kidneys, liver and skin. They do this because certain essential oils have the power to stimulate body systems which may have become sluggish and less than maximally efficient.

What Are Essential Oils?

Basically they are the strong-smelling ingredients found in many plants. They provide the distinctive aroma you get when you bruise a lavender, sage or rosemary leaf, for instance. Most flowers, seeds, grains, roots and resins contain essential oils in minute quantities.

Some of these oils are healing, and some are harmful. Harmful essential oils include wormwood and bitter almond. Healing oils include rosemary, geranium, patchouli, lavender, and sweet almond. Oils from plants become 'essential' after they have been distilled, and the highly concentrated 'essence' is obtained. As very little oil is obtained from each plant, the concentrated form of essential oils is very expensive indeed.

Once the oils have been distilled they are very volatile and will quickly evaporate. This is why you always find aromatherapy oils in dark blue or brown bottles to keep the destructive effect of light away from their contents.

Chemically speaking, these oils are very complicated, and this is where their therapeutic power lies. They are readily absorbed through the skin, and taken up into the bloodstream. Sometimes they can have a very quick effect indeed. I have spoken to some cellulite sufferers who have had to get up off the couch and go to the toilet whilst having the oils rubbed in by an aromatherapist.

Certain oils have a diuretic effect, some are relaxing, while others are stimulating and energizing. Just to give a few examples – clary sage is a powerful relaxant and helps digestion; geranium is an adrenal cortex stimulant and reliever of fluid retention; lavender is calming and soothing; cypress is a powerful astringent; juniper purifies and stimulates the urino-genital tract. Rosemary encourages the lymphatic system to start working properly.

There are literally hundreds of essential oils and it would take years to learn how to use them all properly. But you do not need to be a qualified aromatherapist mixing up mysterious oils to enable them to release their powerful alchemy. Luckily, much of the work has already been done for the cellulite sufferer, so all you have to do is make sure you buy the right kind of oils and use them correctly.

There are two ways of using aromatherapy to combat

cellulite. You can either do it yourself, or you can go to a qualified therapist. Some will find it nicer and perhaps more self-disciplinary to go to a therapist, but it is perfectly possible to use the oils all by yourself to help the cellulite to disappear.

Self Help

There are now a number of special anti-cellulite oils on the market which are based on aromatherapy principles. These are not the highly expensive 'miracle creams' but a mixture of essential oils diluted in the correct carrier oils. You can either buy anti-cellulite oils ready mixed, or make up your own from small bottles of essential oils.

The three main manufacturers of anti-cellulite oils in the UK are **Bodytreats**, **The Body Shop** and **Neal's Yard Apothecary**.

Bodytreats have formulated a twin anti-cellulite pack consisting of two dark-brown bottles, a tiny one and a larger one. The tiny bottle contains 'neat' essential oil for the bath, and the larger one is a dilution of the same oils in a vegetable carrier oil, for massage afterwards. You should put six to ten drops from the small bottle into the bath, but never apply directly to the skin, as it may cause irritation.

Both bottles contain a mixture of rosemary, lavender, geranium and patchouli. The carrier oil in the large bottle is a mixture of grapeseed and wheatgerm oil, which is hand-mixed.

The Body Shop also produces a specific anti-cellulite oil, which is a mixture of lemon, mandarin and apricot essential oils in a sweet almond base. You should massage this in after body brushing and a bath. This oil is not suitable for putting in the bath, as it is specifically a massage oil.

Neal's Yard Apothecary in Covent Garden have a differently formulated anti-cellulite oil, containing lemon, frankincense, juniper, black pepper and sandalwood in a base oil. Their leaflet states that the oil will help to 'eliminate toxins developing in the fatty tissues and in the body'. Black pepper is a very hot essential oil and you may find yourself tingling after massaging in this particular anti-cellulite treatment.

Please see the Appendix for details on how to mix your own anti-cellulite oils.

Use of the Oils

After body brushing in the way described in the previous chapter, shake between six and ten drops of essential oil (*not* the massage oil) into the bath. Lie there, if possible, for about a quarter of an hour, breathing deeply and letting the concentrated oil do its work. As you lie in the bath, knead and pummel the cellulite-heavy areas. You will soon get to know which these are.

Then, after getting out of the bath and drying yourself, massage a small amount of the diluted oil into each thigh, and the buttocks. You can do this with your hands, paying particular attention to the cellulite areas, or with a loofah. Also rub a tiny amount of the oil over your stomach to increase detoxification, and then get dressed. The oils will take about ten minutes to be absorbed completely, and there will be no residual 'oiliness' on your skin after this time. The oils should not spoil or stain clothes if you rub them in sufficiently.

It is best to perform the anti-cellulite treatments either first thing in the morning or, if you don't have time then, in the early evening. Don't do it last thing at night, not because there is anything inherently dangerous in the programme but because the combination of skin brushing, bath and massage will probably keep you awake, as the overall effect is extremely stimulating.

At first you should do the body brushing, aromatherapy and massage every day. Then, after about three or four weeks, use the massage oils every other day. When most of the cellulite has dispersed – and you will know this by your new sleek outline and lack of dimples – use the body brush plus the oils just once or twice a week.

As you progress with the treatment you will probably notice that previously hard areas of thigh and buttock have become soft and flabby. Now, you may think that flab is as bad as cellulite, but actually it's not. This kind of flab is a temporary condition brought about when the fatty cells are emptied of their excess water content. Brisk massage and exercise plus continued use of the aromatherapy oils will tone up the flab, and you will soon notice it firming up.

Do keep the measure handy to measure your thighs. There

will soon be a visible difference, if you apply the oils conscientiously and regularly.

If you do decide to treat your cellulite yourself, make sure you use only the proper aromatherapy oils, or anti-cellulite oils blended on aromatherapy principles. Don't be tempted to spend large sums of money on creams which are supposed to 'improve circulation'. They will not help a cellulite problem to any great extent.

In her article on cellulite in *The Sunday Times* Maggie Drummond wondered what might happen to the fat if these creams worked. Was it shifted elsewhere, she asked, or might it disappear altogether? In any case, she could not understand how the creams could possibly make an iota of difference. 'Do I believe that a contour cream is what it takes for a slimmer, trimmer thigh?' she wrote. 'Pull the other one. It's got gingko biloba tree extract on it.'

In other words, scepticism was absolute. Until it is generally known and accepted that cellulite is a quite different problem from ordinary excess fat, this kind of unhelpful confusion will continue.

Note: although aromatherapy oils are extremely effective at getting rid of cellulite, *they will not work unless you also stick to the diet*. There is not much point in going to all the trouble and expense of aromatherapy treatments if you continue to smoke, drink and eat junk, for as fast as you are getting rid of accumulated toxic wastes, new ones are entering the body.

Going to a Therapist

Women who have huge amounts of cellulite, or fear that they may lack the willpower and motivation to give themselves regular treatments, may be better off going to a qualified therapist who has had proven success in treating cellulite.

When booking up an aromatherapist, ask her to give you the names of people who have already been treated, and speak to them. No reputable therapist will mind putting you in touch with grateful clients – in fact, very many aromatherapists never advertise, but get new customers simply by word of mouth.

When speaking to women who have been successfully treated, ask how long it took, what it cost, and how the treatment progressed. Then, if you feel satisfied, book up six sessions. For most people, this should be enough to get rid of the worst of the problem. However, in my own case, six sessions of extremely hard massage with the oils hardly made any difference and I had to book up more treatments. You will usually be advised to have two treatments a week – they are more effective when coming close together.

Usually the first treatment will consist of a consultation, where the therapist will ask important questions about general health, varicose veins, any pills or medical treatment you may be having. If you have high blood pressure, or any other serious or chronic illness such as a heart condition, asthma, or a recurring skin condition, you should see a therapist rather than attempt to treat the cellulite by yourself. Certain oils are contra-indicated if there are chronic health problems.

The therapist will explain that, however hard she works to pummel away the cellulite deposits, at least sixty per cent of the work must come from you, the patient. You have to make up your mind to stick to the diet, which may consist of nothing but mineral water and fresh fruits for about three days, to begin the detoxifying process. After that, you can gradually add more foods, making sure always that your diet consists mainly of natural wholefoods. You will be much better off if you can manage a completely vegetarian diet, as this is far less toxic than a meat one.

For the actual therapy sessions the practitioner will ask you to take off all your clothes except pants and bra – and will then inspect and assess the cellulite. A vigorous massage session will follow, lasting for about half an hour. If the cellulite is really bad or deep, this massage may hurt. A therapist who has been trained in lymphatic drainage massage will really dig in. You will know when she reaches the cellulite points as there will be a moment of sharp pain. During the initial sessions, you may find your legs are covered in bruises afterwards.

Remember that drastic changes will be taking place inside your body as the cellulite disperses, and these may be accompanied by insomnia, outbreaks of acne, a difference in menstrual patterns, mood changes and negative feelings. You may get colds and flu, catarrh, and headaches. Tissues may be very tender at first.

The worse the cellulite, the more dramatic the changes will be, but all the nasty side effects will disappear before long. As the treatments proceed, you will feel and become quite a different person. Your body image and self-esteem will be raised, and you will certainly notice higher energy levels, as the toxins are released from the system.

My therapist, Frances Clifford, used a mixture of cypress, lavender, juniper berry and clary sage on my cellulite and found that after eight treatments it started moving really quickly. When I first went along, my legs were a solid mass of cellulite, but eventually this was reduced to isolated pockets here and there. These 'pockets' were extremely resistant, as they had probably been there for a very long time, but eventually they too started to disperse.

Removing cellulite can be likened to getting rid of rust, or cleaning up silver that has been neglected for a long time. The longer it has been left, the more difficult the job, but in every case, if you persevere for long enough, the tarnish and rust will go. You just need enough elbow grease and the right rust-dissolving preparation.

As the treatment proceeds, most therapists will keep quite detailed case notes, to enable them to keep a check on progress. A reputable therapist will be able to tell you whether you have a water retention problem in addition to the cellulite. Usually, though, you will know this because water retention means thick, spongy ankles. There are, of course, aromatherapy treatments which can combat this problem but they are slightly different. For one thing, the type of massage used will be far lighter and gentler.

All aromatherapists have different ways of treating cellulite, though the overall understanding of the condition is the same. Patricia Davis uses a combination of detoxifying, hormone-balance and lymphatic-system-stimulating oils, plus those which have mildly diurectic properties. She says that as the treatment will possibly need to be continued over several weeks or even months, depending on the extent of the cellulite, it is important to vary the oils. As with any medicines, the body gets used to the same oils after a time, and they lose their effectiveness.

Patricia usually begins treatment with a combination of geranium and rosemary in equal proportions, and incorporates a small amount of black pepper, juniper and fennel. She also suggests that clients should drink fennel tea several times a day.

Another aromatherapist, Danièle Ryman, uses a mixture of cypress, lavender and lemon, and advises drinking sage and vervain teas.

Also, as people are themselves very individual, they may react differently to the oils. I found that the Bodytreats anti-cellulite oils were extremely stimulating, and kept me awake if I used them too late at night. A good therapist will discover the range of oils which are just right for your particular condition, general health status, age, skin type and temperament.

Whether you decide to enlist the help of a therapist or go it alone it is important to regard cellulite removal as a medical treatment, in much the same way as you would approach getting rid of acne, eczema, migraine, or any other chronic condition which makes you feel miserable and depressed.

All aromatherapists recognize that there is a significant stress component in cellulite, and that the condition is far more likely to form at times of tension and anxiety. This is why it is very common for cellulite to be laid down when young women first leave home to go to university or college, embark on a disastrous love affair, have to tackle difficult exams or projects at work, or give up a career to bring up children. Any prolonged stressful event can encourage cellulite to form, as all poisons are more readily held in the system when there is a state of stress.

A good aromatherapist will recognize this, and combine the vigorous massage with a calm-down massage before the treatment finishes. The total effect of the treatments is to leave you in a calmer and more confident state.

Perhaps these sound like large claims to make for a treatment which appears to consist simply of having a variety of fragrant and exotic oils rubbed into your legs. But to my mind the proof of the pudding is in the eating. Many, many women in this country have removed their cellulite by this means, and are successfully keeping it off.

CHAPTER SEVEN

THE BENEFITS OF MASSAGE

Massage is the final important ingredient of any success-ful cellulite-removing regime. If you are carrying out a self-help programme you should always make sure you massage the oils in well after a bath, rather than just rubbing them in.

First of all, pour a little massage oil – about a teaspoonful – into the palm of your hand, and rub it slightly into your hands. You should never pour any oils directly onto the skin. Then with long stroking movements start at the ankle and work up to the knee and thigh. Use both hands and make sure the movements are gentle but firm. This type of massage encourages circulation and can stimulate blood flow.

A good type of massage for cellulite-laden areas is **knead-ing**, which is also known by masseurs as *pétrissage*. For this, you have to pretend you are kneading a loaf of bread as you pick up the flesh and squeeze it, applying as much pressure as you can. It is rather like pinching huge areas of flesh.

After doing this, you can go back and pinch up the flesh in the very worst of the cellulite areas. You will soon get to know which these are.

Another useful movement for cellulite sufferers is **rolling**.

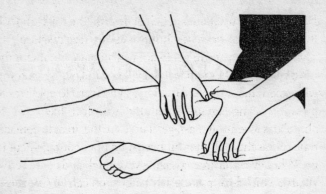

kneading

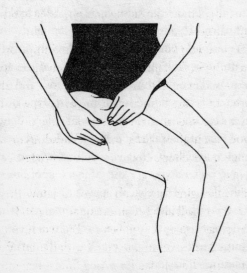

rolling

Here, you pick up about an inch of flesh on the thigh and roll the flesh to break down the lumpy deposits (see diagram).

After a time you will get to know which areas contain the most cellulite. They will feel ridgy, hard and grainy, and you will experience a ripply sensation as you learn to apply more pressure. Long-ingrained cellulite will feel like rows of chipolatas when you massage. These are the areas to concentrate on, as the cellulite will need a lot of encouragement to go. Whenever you are massaging your thigh and come across an area which feels particularly tender you can be sure this is where the cellulite is at its worst.

Once you feel you have got to know your cellulite, you can dig at it with your thumb, using as much pressure as you are able to. Now you have embarked on an anti-cellulite programme, any kind of kneading and pinching and pounding will only do good.

Make sure you knead and pound the lumpy areas when you are lying in the bath, especially if you have shaken in a few drops of concentrated essential oils. You can also knead and wring the spare flesh at any time of day – whenever you have a few moments of privacy. From now on any kind of attention, such as stroking, rolling, kneading or wringing, will have good effects and you will soon start seeing the difference.

Daily massaging helps you to get to know the cellulite areas, and you will also become acquainted with your whole body in a way you never did before. But when you pummel away at the lumpy areas, don't do it with hatred. Very many women – myself included for a long time – feel only disgust when they look down at their thighs, and start hating their legs. When massaging, you should treat the thighs with loving care, reminding yourself that you are doing your very best for them, to enable them to lose the rubbish the fat cells have held for so long. In the same way that some people speak to plants, therapists often advise their clients to start talking to their cellulite, and to try and visualize it seeping out of fatty cells as they knead and pound away at the bulgy areas. It may sound ridiculous at first, but visualization has become a very popular therapy for cancer patients in America. Some clinics advise patients to use their imagination and see the tumours shrinking as they concentrate on their cancer.

Now, I'm not for one minute suggesting that cellulite is a problem on the same level as cancer, but it is unwanted and unhealthy just the same. Visualization can be very effective when you are massaging, as it helps you to concentrate hard on the cellulite areas, rather than going off into a day dream.

Whenever you are alone, watching television, or otherwise relaxing, put your legs in the air one at a time, and gently stroke up them, starting at the ankle and going right up to the hip joint. This encourages the lymphatic system to become more active, and also helps toxic wastes to start draining away.

It is the regularity of the massage which makes the difference. At first, when the cellulite is very bad, you should make sure you do it every single day. The order is: body brushing, bath (with drops of essential oils), then massaging in the oils. At first, it may seem extremely self-indulgent to spend so much time on yourself every day, but the rewards will soon be noticed in disappearing cellulite.

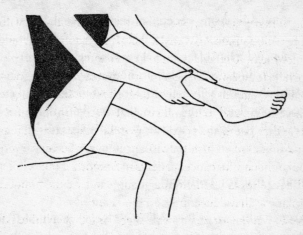

During the past few years, there has been an enormous upsurge of interest in massage techniques. It is now at last being accepted that all types of massage, from gentle stroking to hard pounding and pummelling, can have enormous beneficial effects on the whole system. Like aromatherapy, massage used to be regarded rather as a self-indulgent beauty treatment, something which was medically neither here nor there.

Now we know differently. Pioneering masseuses such as Clare Maxwell-Hudson have shown that the ancient art of massage can be at least as effective as much modern medicine, and can bring about dramatic changes in the body. American masseuse Ouida West says in her book, *The Magic of Massage*, 'I define massage as any touch that is capable of evoking a change in the body. Even the lightest touch, when properly executed, may effectively stimulate circulation or alter the flow of energy within the body.'

Among the many benefits of massage Ouida West lists: improvement of self-esteem; relief of neck and shoulder tension; reduction of fat stored in the tissues; dilation of blood vessels to improve circulation; improvement of digestion, assimilation and elimination. Kidney function can be increased, and the lymphatic system can be flushed out by elimination of toxins and waste through massage.

Take Time for Yourself

Women who live by themselves are lucky when embarking on an anti-cellulite regime, because they can please themselves what they eat, when they massage, and when they have their bath. Those who are married, have a family, or share a flat may not be so fortunate, because it has to be admitted that those you live with will, on the whole, resent the time you take for yourself. You may also have to cope with comments such as: 'but you're quite thin enough as you are', or 'but I *like* your legs like that'. This type of remark is most often passed by the man in one's life. Men can particularly get annoyed when the women in their life go off and massage and pummel their thighs.

The strength of mind needed to combat cellulite successfully should never be over-estimated. You just have to make up your mind not to hear these remarks, and carry on, even while others may tell you – usually without knowing the first thing about the subject themselves – that it's a complete waste of time and money. I know from experience that you have to be completely singleminded when deciding to banish cellulite. Like an unwelcome guest, it never wants to go, and will take up permanent squatter's rights in your body whenever it can. You just have to regard it in the same way as household dust and dirt – something you must continually struggle to keep down.

Daily massage is really essential, so do make sure you make time to include it in your general routine. Occasional pummellings and kneadings are not enough.

Although very many massage books on the market speak enthusiastically about people learning to do massage for each other, I have very strong doubts about whether this really works. Mostly, people are encouraged to massage each other for sexual or intimate reasons, and with cellulite-removal this is the last thing on your mind. You are carrying out a self-help medical treatment, not indulging in sexual foreplay. For this reason, I would say that it is not a good idea for a husband, boyfriend or lover to try and help you get rid of your cellulite. For one thing, most of them couldn't care a hoot whether you have cellulite or not, and for another, the intimate kind of stroking needed could soon take a sexual turn.

If you have friends who are professional masseurs, or who have taken courses, then that is a different thing. But I can't think it would be a good idea to entrust your body to somebody who doesn't know what they are doing. It's far better to do it by yourself, and take responsibility for yourself.

Going to a Therapist

If you are considering going to a professional, make sure you choose somebody who is qualified to practise both aromatherapy and lymphatic drainage. It is important to ask about the lymphatic draining, because this will be your clue that the therapist really can help you. If you get a confused silence on the end of the phone when you ask your local aromatherapist about this kind of massage, then don't book her up. Also ask, of course, about the nutritional aspects, as no massage alone, however tough, can disperse cellulite. It is essential that your therapist should understand exactly what cellulite is.

Lymphatic Drainage Massage

This is a highly specialized technique whereby the masseuse activates the main lymph nodes in order to get them working again. She does this by pressing on the lymph points all over your body and applying pressure to them. Although you would probably need to go to a professional to get a proper lymphatic drainage, you can easily learn for yourself where the main lymph nodes are, and press these after you have finished the kneading and pounding massage.

The diagram opposite shows where the main points are – under the armpits, in the thoracic duct between the breasts, in the lumbar region, behind the knees. It won't take long to learn where these are, and touching them will definitely help the lymphatic system to get working properly again.

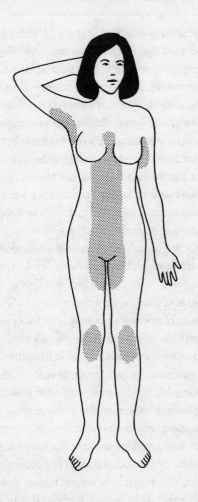

Some people find that when the body is really overloaded with toxic and waste matter the lymph nodes feel tender. If this is the case with you, don't give up, but keep applying gentle pressure until the tenderness ceases. As you carry on with the regime, you will find that the nodes become less tender. Tenderness in these regions means that there is a blockage, and it may take time for this to be released.

Those who are going to a therapist should always say when they feel any pain or tenderness in any area whatever. You can't expect her to be a mind reader, although an experienced therapist will be aware of possible tender points.

A professional anti-cellulite massage will usually take between half and three-quarters of an hour, and the therapist will concentrate only on the cellulite areas and the lymphatic points. She will not usually give you a general massage, and she will not touch your back or your front. You can of course, if you like, ask for a general massage, but this is a different kind of treatment.

The advantage of going to a therapist is that an objective check will be kept on your progress, but don't imagine that all is lost if you cannot find anybody suitable in your area. At the time of writing, there are not many people trained in this form of massage who have also studied the vital nutritional and dietary aspects, which is one of the reasons I'm writing this book! Once you have the information at your fingertips, and can understand exactly what cellulite is and what is needed to remove it, you can effectively become your own therapist.

Most professionals finish up by stroking the abdomen gently in circular movements. This aids the digestive system,

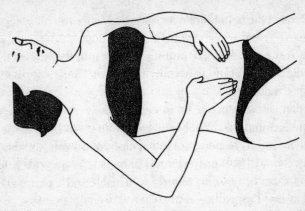

and also helps waste products to disperse. It is easy enough to do this for yourself, using a tiny trace of oil. Make sure the movements are extremely gentle here.

When a professional massage has been completed, you will usually be asked to lie still on the couch for a few minutes to collect yourself. Lymphatic drainage massage can be very hard and tough, and you may feel slightly faint if you get up instantly. If you are doing your own massage, take a tip from the professionals, and lie down for a little while after you have finished. I can guarantee that you will feel quite wonderful when you get up.

The timing of daily self-massage is important. You probably won't have time to do it properly first thing in the morning, and last thing at night the whole exercise can be far too stimulating. So the optimum time is early evening, before supper. If you can get into the habit of performing the anti-cellulite massage at this time you will definitely have renewed energy for the evening, and will not be tempted to fill yourself up with snacks and junk foods.

One of the benefits of massage is that, after you have been cosseting and caring for your body on the outside in this way, you feel much less like putting rubbish into the inside. By massaging yourself, you learn to respect your body, both inside and out.

You will also notice other benefits from regular massage with essential oils. Your skin and clothes will become delicately impregnated with the fragrance of the oils, and also your skin will become softer and smoother. You are likely to have fewer headaches, to feel less irritable and touchy, and less stressed generally.

Anything which reduces stress is to be recommended because, of course, there is a major stress element in the development of cellulite. The less tense and anxious you are, the less cellulite will be formed. This is not just some airy-fairy notion but a scientifically acknowledged fact. When the mind is tense and anxious extra stress hormones (adrenalin) are released into the system, and stay there. The more chronic the stress, the greater the release of adrenalin and the greater, eventually, the build-up of toxic wastes.

Digestion, elimination and circulation are all adversely affected by mental stress. We are only just learning – or appreciating – how closely linked the mind and body are, and how intimately the feedback principle operates. Whatever affects the mind will soon reverberate in the body, and vice versa. Massage is a potent means of unstressing the system, and thus counteracting the production of excess adrenalin.

As we know, the formation of cellulite is basically an elimination problem, so anything which helps body systems to return to normal will also aid reduction of these wastes.

What About Exercise?

As most cellulite sufferers know only too well, no amount of exercise will shift even a millimetre of cellulite. This doesn't mean you shouldn't be physically active, of course, only that you should not even begin to rely on exercise to get rid of the lumps and bumps.

We know, of course, that the formation of cellulite is associated with leading a sedentary life, which in turn means that circulation is likely to be poor. So exercise can very much help to *prevent* cellulite. If you look at leading female athletes, such as Zola Budd, Mary Decker Slaney and marathon runner Ingrid Christiansen, you will notice that not one of them has even the tiniest trace of cellulite. All have legs which look as if they are made from the lightest and best-tempered steel, with not an ounce of flab or spare flesh. Because these women have been athletes ever since they were children, it is unlikely that cellulite ever had a chance to lay itself down.

The time to embark on exercise is once the cellulite has started to disappear. As soon as you begin an anti-cellulite programme, you should make up your mind to become as physically active as possible. This means walking instead of taking a bus or the lift at work and going for a swim whenever possible. Any gentle, rhythmic form of exercise will help to keep circulation moving, which is what you are aiming at.

Once you are left with residual flab, after the worst of the cellulite has made its exit, you can do the tried and tested bicycling in the air, copy somebody like Lizzie Webb on breakfast television, or book up keep-fit classes at a local gym.

Local-authority-run keep-fit and conditioning classes are extremely cheap, and usually very good.

Yoga exercises will also firm up flabby muscles, if you are that way inclined. Although yoga classes will help to put a long-misused body back into alignment, the movements are too slow and sustained to be of enormous help in muscle toning. Yoga positions will certainly help you to find out where the cellulite-laden areas are, and enable you to realize where stiffness and lack of suppleness lie, but they are not specifically designed to firm up the flab left when cellulite makes its exit.

The good thing about yoga positions, or *asanas* as they are known, is that by doing them – or at least attempting them – you get to know and respect your own body. The other valuable aspect of yoga is that it is not harmful in any way, as perhaps aerobics or California-stretch-type classes might be.

What you should never do is attempt a vigorous work-out if you have been completely sedentary for years on end. This is as much a shock to the system as a drastically altered diet – and the body may not be able to cope. Many women find that, once they have got rid of the worst of the cellulite, they have a far more positive attitude to their bodies and no longer fear putting on a leotard or joining an exercise class. This is good – but don't be tempted to overdo it at first. Apart from anything else, you'll never keep it up. It is far better to start with a very gentle exercise regime intended for beginners, and then gradually become more vigorous as your body can take it.

There are now many multi-gyms around the country, and also all kinds of exercise machines you can buy for yourself.

The Benefits of Massage

The great majority of people use exercise bikes and the like for a short time and then become bored and forget about them. If you suspect this is you, don't be tempted to spend vast sums of money on expensive home gyms. It would be far better for you to attend weekly sessions at a commercial gym, where your progress will be monitored.

Of course, after you have completed an anti-cellulite programme, your body and general health will be far better than before, and you will probably feel much more like doing exercise. To be effective, any exercise has to be regular, and you will never keep it up unless you enjoy it. You should walk or swim at least three times a week and, ideally, go to keep-fit classes twice a week. Exercise experts have worked out that, in order to do any good, your chosen form of exercise should be practised at least three times a week, and for at least twenty minutes at a time. Any less, and you might as well not bother.

However, if you get rid of the cellulite first, by being conscientious about the regime outlined in this book, and then complete the good work by the right kind of exercise, you will – I promise you – be rewarded by the kind of figure and good health you had never previously dreamed possible.

It happened to me. And if I, as a lifelong exercise-hater and self-indulgent soul, can get rid of cellulite after more than twenty years, so can you.

PREPARING YOUR OWN ANTI-CELLULITE OILS

You should always match up bath oils to massage oils when embarking on anti-cellulite treatments. Essential oils which are good to put in the bath include lemon, rosemary, geranium, patchouli, cypress or juniper. These are all equally effective, and can be bought as single oils from any supplier of aromatherapy products such as Neal's Yard, Culpeper, Bodytreats, or The Body Shop.

Lemon has an alkalizing effect on body systems, cypress is good for those who have any problems with their veins, and juniper is particularly effective for people who smoke or who have to travel or work in crowded, smoky environments.

You should shake six to ten drops of the essential oil into the bath and relax in the water for about fifteen minutes. After you have dried yourself, massage in the massage oils. These can easily be made by filling a 100 ml bottle – it should be opaque and dark – with the base or carrier oil, and then shaking about thirty drops of the essential oil into this.

The base, or carrier, oil that you use is important. It should be pure vegetable oil such as sweet almond, apricot kernel, avocado (very rich), grapeseed, hazelnut or sunflower. Ordinary kitchen cooking oil will do so long as it is not blended, and is cold-pressed. If it is cold-pressed, it will say so on the label. You can use olive oil if you like, although this is rather strong-smelling. But it works perfectly well as a carrier oil.

Remember that the massage action is as important as the oil itself, so rub it in as hard as you can.

Some essential oils are not suitable for anti-cellulite treatments. These include all the spice oils and most of the flower oils, which have no effect whatever. The best ones to use are the herb oils or the tree oils, as these work to improve circulation and are also invigorating and toning. Each essential oil, like each herb, has a specific quality and not all are equally good.

You can also burn oils to inhale the fragrance. Oil burners can be bought from most craftshops and fill the air with a wonderful fragrance which has potent de-stressing qualities. Lavender, which helps to take acid out of the system, is good for burning whenever you feel tense and anxious, but any of the oils listed above will do the same job. Six drops are all you need to release the fragrance. This can be done whenever you don't have time for a bath, and should be done as often as you can, as one of the causes of cellulite is, of course, undue stress.

Do remember whenever embarking on anti-cellulite treatments never to sit with crossed legs. This cuts off circulation and encourages cellulite to form. Try to get into the habit of sitting with legs straight, and with ankles higher than hips whenever possible.

IMPORTANT: You should never use the same oils for more

than two to three weeks at a time, as they lose their potency once the body gets used to them. In this, they are exactly like any other drug. For rapid effect, change your oils frequently. For instance, if you use cypress for the first three weeks, change to rosemary for the next three weeks. The body likes to be surprised and stimulated.

BIBLIOGRAPHY

Campion, Kitty: A Woman's Herbal, Century, 1987

Davies, Dr Stephen and Stewart, Dr Alan: Nutritional Medicine, Pan, 1987

Davis, Patricia: Aromatherapy: An A–Z, C. W. Daniel, 1988

Gray, Dr Robert: The Colon Health Handbook, Rockridge Publishing Company, California, 1983

Hepper, Camilla: Herbal Cosmetics, Thorsons, 1987

Kenton, Leslie: The Joy of Beauty, Century, 1983

Kenton, Leslie, and Kenton, Susannah: Raw Energy Recipes, Century, 1985

Maxwell-Hudson, Clare: The Complete Book of Massage, Dorling Kindersley, 1988

Maxwell-Hudson, Clare: Your Health and Beauty Book, Macdonald, 1979

Maxwell-Hudson, Clare: The Natural Beauty Book, Macdonald, 1983

Ryman, Danièle: The Aromatherapy Handbook, Century, 1984

Soltanoff, Dr Jack: Natural Healing, Warner Books (USA), 1988

Bibliography

Tisserand, Robert: *The Art of Aromatherapy*,
   C. W. Daniel, 1977
Tisserand, Robert: *Aromatherapy for Everyone*, Penguin,
   1988
Valnet, Dr Jean: *The Practice of Aromatherapy*,
   C. W. Daniel, 1982
West, Ouida: *The Magic of Massage*, Century, 1983
Wright, Brian: *Cleansing the Colon*, Green Press, 1987
Wright, Celia: *The Wright Diet*, Piatkus, 1986

USEFUL ADDRESSES

Aromatherapy courses

The London School of
   Aromatherapy,
PO Box 780
London NW6 5EQ

Also has a list of trained
aromatherapists in the UK and
other parts of the world.
Principal: Patricia Davis.

The International Federation
   of Aromatherapists
46 Dalkeith Road
Dulwich
London SE21 8LS

This organization has a list of
accredited schools and
colleges, as well as individual
aromatherapists. It is a
registered charity.

Aromatherapy Oils

Bodytreats Ltd
15 Approach Road
Raynes Park
London SW20 8BA

Norman and Germaine Rich
2 Coval Gardens
London SW14 7DG

Micheline Arcier
   Aromatherapy
7 William Street
London SW1

Neal's Yard Apothecary
Neal's Yard
Covent Garden
London WC2

Branches of The Body Shop

Branches of Holland & Barrett

Body brushes

Available from:

Green Farm Nutrition Centre
Burwash Common
East Sussex TN19 7LA

Green Farm also publish a
specialized anti-cellulite diet.

Branches of The Body Shop

Kitty Campion
The Natural Health and
Iridology Centre
19 Park Terrace
Tunstall
Stoke on Trent
Staffs ST6 6PB

Kitty will also help with
anti-cellulite treatments.

Nutritional Information

For advice on detoxifying and
cleansing diets, contact Green
Farm Nutrition Centre, as
above, or:

The Institute for Optimum
Nutrition
5 Jerdan Place
London SW6 1BE

The Nutritional Advisory
Service
PO Box 268
Hove,
East Sussex BN3 1R3

*Massage Courses and
Information*

The Clare Maxwell-Hudson
School of Massage
PO Box 457
London NW2 4BR

Note: please enclose large
s.a.e. when writing to any of
these addresses.

INDEX

Index

Index

Nobody can write Forbidden Fantasies like Cara Summers!

Of *Led Into Temptation*

"Sensationally sensual…this tale of a forbidden, guilt-ridden love is a delight. Brimming with diverse, compelling characters, scorching-hot love scenes, romance and even a ghost, this story is unforgettable."
—*Romancejunkies.com*

"This deliciously naughty fantasy takes its time heating up, but it's worth the wait!…"
—*RT Book Reviews*

Of *Taken Beyond Temptation*

"Great characters with explosive chemistry, a fun intrigue-flavored plot and a high degree of sensuality add up to an excellent read!…"
—*RT Book Reviews*

"Filled with intrigue, mystery, humor, sizzling-\t love scenes, a well-matched couple, a surprise \nding and a ghost, this story is unforgettable and definitely a winner."
—*Romancejunkies.com*

Of *Twice the Temptation*

"ll written!… Fans will be delighted to see their favorites return for brief appearances…"
—*RT Book Reviews*

"Cara Summers has penned two tales in *Twice the Temptation* wh
on